Colour Atlas of
Micro-Oto-Neurosurgical
Procedures

*To our wives and children
so patiently accepting
their husbands and fathers*

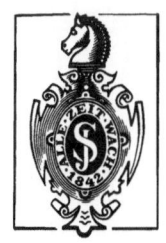

Vittorio Colletti M.D.   James E. Benecke Jr. M.D.

Colour Atlas of Micro-Oto-Neurosurgical Procedures

Foreword by - W. F. House M.D. and V. Ricci M.D.

Introduction by W. F. House
With 112 figures.

Springer-Verlag London Ltd.

Vittorio Colletti, M.D.
Associate Professor of Oto-Rhino-Laryngology, ENT Department, Faculty of Medicine - University of Verona, Italy.

William F. House M.D.
Clinical Professor, University of Southern California, School of Medicine. Otologic Medical Group Inc. - House Ear Institute, Los Angeles, California U.S.A.

James E. Benecke Jr. M.D.
Clinical Assistant Professor, University of Southern California, School of Medicine. Otologic Medical Group Inc. - House Ear Institute. Los Angeles, California, U.S.A.

Vincenzo Ricci M.D.
Professor of Oto-Rhino-Laryngology, ENT Department, Faculty of Medicina, University of Verona, Italy

Front cover illustrations, see pages 35, 48, 66, 94

ISBN 978-1-4471-3791-7

British Library Cataloguing in Publication Data
Colletti, V. Vittorio, *1943-*
    Colour atlas of micro oto neurological procedures.
    1. Man. Nervous system. Surgery
    I. Title   II. Benecke, J. (James), *1952-*
    617'.48
ISBN 978-1-4471-3791-7   ISBN 978-1-4471-3789-4 (eBook)
DOI 10.1007/978-1-4471-3789-4

Library of Congress Cataloging-in-Publication Data
Colletti, V.
    Colour atlas fo micro-oto-neurosurgical procedure.
    Bibliography: p.
    Includes index.
    1. Ear--Surgery--Atlases.   2. Microsurgery--Atlases.
I. Benecke, James E., 1952-   II.Title.
(DNLM: 1. Ear-surgery--atlases.   2. Microsurgery--methods--atlases. WV 17 C698c)
RF126.C65 1988   617.8'059   88-35947
ISBN 978-1-4471-3791-7

© 1989 Springer-Verlag London
Originally published by Springer-Verlag Berlin Heidelberg New York Tokyo in 1989
Softcover reprint of the hardcover 1st edition 1989

Typeset by Byland, Verona - Italy
Photogravure by Eurografica, Verona - Italy

Contents

Foreword

Modern microsurgical techniques have opened up a new horizon for the otoneurosurgeon. This volume is a very important contribution to the student who is learning these surgical approaches. Surgical otoneurology has now passed the infancy stage, but is still an adolescent. As more otologists and neurosurgeons become skilled in this type of surgery, new and better approaches will evolve. Certainly there needs to be much better management of the carotid artery as it passes through the temporal bone. Better techniques to preserve the IX, X, and XI nerves in the jugular bulb area should be developed, and more delicate procedures for management of lesions inside the cochlea and vestibular labyrinth should be developed. As our diagnostic techniques have improved, particularly through imaging, surgical techniques to match the improved diagnostic techniques will emerge. For future otoneurologists who are prepared, many problems involving the temporal bone that are now considered untreatable will be successfully managed for very grateful patients. The purpose of this text is to familiarize the otoneurosurgeon with the anatomy of the temporal bone, skull base, infratemporal fossa, and cerebellopontine angle. This anatomy will be taught by demonstrating surgical procedures.

This atlas which is an example of cooperation between the schools of Los Angeles and Verona will permit the reader to rehearse otoneurosurgical procedures in the laboratory, and, when the techniques have been mastered, apply the various approaches in the treatment of inner ear and skull base lesions.

William F. House M.D.
Vincenzo Ricci M.D.

Introduction

Otoneurology dates back to 1914 when Bárány won the Nobel Prize in Medicine for his monumental contributions to the evaluation and study of the vestibular system. Otoneurology remained largely a study of the vestibular system until microsurgical procedures opened up vast new possibilities for the treatment of otoneurological clinical problems. It was during the last months of my Residency in 1956 that I first met Professor Wullstein of Würzburg, Germany. He was on a tour of the United States and brought with him the first Zeiss operating microscope I had ever seen, and also some motion pictures that he had taken by mounting the motion picture camera on one of the eyepieces, while he operated through the other. Those movies absolutely stunned me. Seeing the middle ear and mastoid structures through the microscope gave me the same thrill that I experienced years later when seeing live television shots of the moonscape being taken by astronauts, and I became a devoted temporal bone explorer.

Fortunately, I had an abundant supply of cadaver material available at the Los Angeles County Hospital morgue and a wife who was an R.N. and who was willing to work with me nights and week-ends, helping with instrumentation. Working on fresh cadavers was valuable because it forced me always to look at the temporal bone through potential surgical approaches. Each dissection would start with an incision, and using actual surgical instrumentation, I would end up several hours later at some point in the temporal bone. I explored the course of the facial nerve in its entirety from the brain stem out into the face, dissected all of the middle ear structures, the eustachian tube, cochlea, vestibular system, internal auditory canal and the petrous apex. I looked at these same structures from above the temporal bone through the middle fossa, as well from below, coming up from the neck structures. As the months passed I found myself spending the first hour or hour and a half of each dissection session getting through the cortex and mastoid of the temporal bone, and I wondered if there was some way this could be accomplished with more dispatch so that I could spend more time dissecting the deeper structures.I was following the technical procedures I had learned from my brother, Howard House, which were started by Lempert and which required that whenever drilling, two hands were used to steady the dental handpiece, and after a small amount of bone was removed, the wound was irrigated and then suctioned. This procedure was repeated many, many times while going through the cortex and mastoid cells.

As a dentist in the Navy, I had worked with various irrigation systems, high speed handpieces and the newly emerging technology of diamond stones for cutting the enamel and dentin of tooth structures. It occurred to me that application of some of this technology to temporal bone surgery would be very valuable. I abandoned holding the handpiece with two hands, since I had never done that as a dentist. One hand was used for the handpiece and the other usually for a mirror. I worked out the irrigation suction techniques where the wound could be flooded by decreasing the suction by opening the thumb hole on the irrigation, and then the wound cleared by closing the thumb hole. This greatly speeded the temporal bone dissection, and I actually found it much safer because the bone dust was removed from the mastoid as it was being produced by the cutting burr. I also found that utilization of this irrigation suction technique, along with diamond stones which I obtained from dental supply houses, made for more accurate and delicate bone removal, particularly around structures such as the facial nerve. I also found that there was a great advantage in using diamond stones since they would cut with the burr rotating either clockwise or counterclockwise. In this way the burr could be selectively rotated so that there would be less tendency to catch an edge and injure important temporal bone structures.

Another important opportunity in my early years of practice was that stapes surgery, which had been pioneered by Rosen and John Shea, was in full swing. Since I was associated in practice with Howard, who previously had had a very large practice dealing with fenestration surgery and was now very busy with stapes procedures, he was more than willing to allow me to take care of the chronic ear problems. Wullstein had pioneered tympanoplasty and had popularized five different types of tympanoplasty, all based on reconstructing the middle ear, but avoiding the reconstruction of the ossicular chain. All of these tympanoplasty procedures, with the exception of the Type I, which was a myringoplasty procedure, involved creating a mastoid cavity, and then placing a graft over the middle ear to increase sound transmission to the oval window. In performing these procedures I found that, while the early results were quite encouraging in terms of maintaining or improving the patient's hearing, all too often a mastoid cavity infection would occur and this would then destroy the graft. I found myself doing many revisions of these procedures. During this time there was much in the literature, and reports at meetings, about filling the cavity with muscle flaps and other tissues in order to avoid the mastoid cavity, but none of these seemed to be very satisfactory since the muscle would tend to atrophy, or whatever other materials were placed in the cavity would ultimately be rejected. More and more it seemed to me that the only real answer was to develop ways of cleaning out all of the infected tissue and cholesteatoma, while leaving the posterior canal wall intact so that a cavity would no longer be a constant problem for the patient. I found that by going through what I decided to call the facial recess area the infected tissue and cholesteatoma could indeed be totally removed. Since I was now violating the age-old principle of temporal bone surgery, which was to open up the mastoid and middle ear spaces so that they could freely drain, it was now necessary to do a very meticulous removal of cholesteatoma and granulation and thus have the mastoid and middle ear heal as a primary healing, rather than to continue to drain.

New problems also arose in that I now found it better to place the graft in the normal eardrum position. This required reconstruction of the ossicular chain. There was more and more interest in this, and of course many different techniques for reconstruction were tried at the time and published by many authors. It was also found that the graft would retract if the middle ear and mastoid were not properly aerated, and so the principles of reconstruction of the ossicular chain and aeration of the middle ear and mastoid became firmly established. Over the first few years of practice, chronic ear procedures had allowed me to become thoroughly familiar with temporal bone surgery and to perfect the techniques that would allow very meticulous surgical dissection.

It was through my observations of patients with otosclerosis that I backed into the first surgical otoneurological procedures. Fenestration surgery had only been performed on patients with essentially normal bone conduction. However, stapes surgery with its possibility of completely closing the air-bone gap extended the benefits of surgery to a much wider range of patients with otosclerosis, namely, those who had varying degrees of sensorineural hearing loss, along with the stapes fixation.

I became interested in why so many patients with otosclerosis had an accompanying sensorineural hearing loss. Indeed, I saw a number of patients in practice who had been patients of Howard's for many years, and could see the progressive sensorineural hearing loss that many of these patients exhibited. In a review of the literature, particularly the volumes summarizing otosclerosis literature published by the American Otologic Society, I found a number of articles indicating that one of the theories for this sensorineural hearing loss was due to a focus of otosclerosis occurring just above the labyrinth and lateral end of the internal auditory canal. This focus was believed to be causing pressure on the VIII nerve, thus causing the increasing sensorineural hearing loss.

I reasoned that if we could surgically remove this otosclerotic focus then perhaps we could take the pressure off the VIII nerve and reverse or stop the progression of the sensorineural hearing loss. June and I again returned to the dissection room and I began a series of dissections from above the temporal bone through the middle cranial fossa. The problem was to be able to unroof the internal auditory canal without damage to the facial nerve or to the structures of the inner ear. The key was to find the greater superficial petrosal nerve, follow this back to the geniculate ganglion, and then follow the facial nerve on down to the internal auditory canal. Over a period of many months I performed this dissection numerous times, and working with Jack Urban, I worked out some early retractors for the temporal lobe. I recruited a neurosurgeon, Dr. Ted Kurze, into this effort since it was a combined intracranial temporal bone procedure. Ted was to elevate the temporal lobe and locate the greater superficial petrosal, and from there I was to complete the middle fossa approach to unroofing the internal auditory canal. On August 1st, 1958, we did our first middle fossa procedure on a patient who essentially had a total loss from advanced otosclerosis. I remember this date quite well because it was June's birthday and she spent that birthday in the operating room with me on this procedure. Unfortunately, this patient, and several others on whom I attempted to improve hearing, did not improve their hearing postoperatively. These procedures, however, demonstrated that we could locate the facial nerve and carefully dissect it in the internal auditory canal. We could see the vestibular nerves and it occurred to me that these procedures might make it possible for us to remove acoustic neuromas and save the facial nerve. At that time all acoustic neuroma surgery completely destroyed the facial nerve while removing the tumor.

Working with a neurosurgeon, Dr. Jack Doyle, techniques were worked out to dissect the labyrinth down to the jugular bulb from the middle fossa approach, and to isolate the facial nerve and remove the tumor through the middle fossa with the patient in a sitting position. It soon became obvious that a better approach would be to go through the mastoid and labyrinth to the internal auditory canal, and thus the translabyrinthine approach was developed.

Today, all parts of the temporal bone and cerebellopontine angle are readily accessible by many different routes. These approaches have opened up vast new treatment possibilities for a whole array of problems involving the facial nerve, the balance system, the hearing mechanisms, and the structures of the jugular bulb and petrous apex.

William F. House M.D.

I. INCISIONS FOR OTO-NEUROLOGICAL SURGERY

Adequate exposure is essential for approaching the cerebellopontine (CP) angle, petrous apex, and clivus through the temporal bone. This begins with the skin incision which must be properly located to afford access to the mastoid cortex and lateral subocciput, or to the petrous apex.

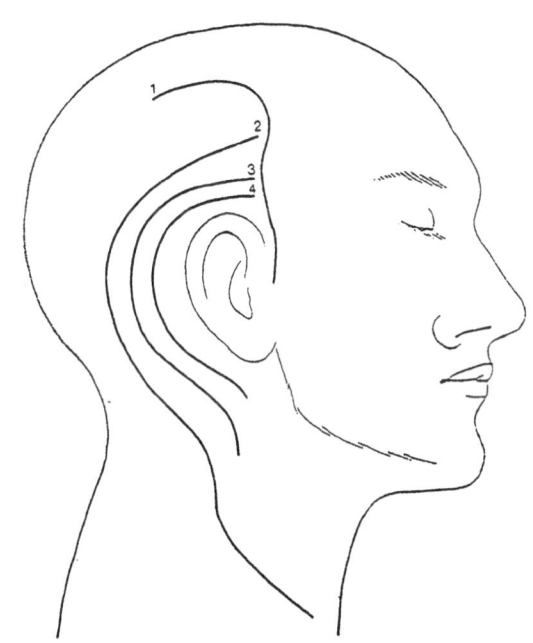

A. Patient draped for oto-neurological surgery.

B. Incisions for middle fossa and for infratemporal fossa procedures will be described in the specific chapters.

C. Incision for translabyrinthine, retrolabyrinthine and transcochlear procedures is placed at least 2.5 cm behind the postauricular sulcus.

D. For retrosigmoid procedures the incision must be carried inferiorly into the upper neck for a distance of 3 cm below the mastoid tip.

1. INCISIONS FOR OTO-NEUROLOGICAL PROCEDURES:

1. Middle fossa	*2. Infratemporal*
3. Retrosigmoid	*4. Translabyrinthine and retrolabyrinthine.*

E. The incision can be made with the cutting current of the electrocautery device as long as the tip of the device is kept moving.

F. Cutting cephalad through the temporalis muscle as depicted in the photograph allows for easy reflection of the muscle out of the field.

G. A sharp elevator is used to elevate soft tissues off the mastoid cortex and lateral subocciput. The spine of Henle is identified and the skin of the external auditory canal is not violated.

H. Large self-retaining retractors are placed into the incision.

Summary: *Make sure that the incision is not placed too close to the postauricular sulcus. The more surface area of temporal bone that can be exposed, the easier the access to deep structures.*

II. COMPLETE SIMPLE MASTOIDECTOMY

The complete simple mastoidectomy is the basic building block for almost all oto-neurosurgical procedures. Adequate bone removal during this step of the surgery assures easier access to deeper structures.

A. The dissection begins posterior to the spine of Henle. Using the largest cutting burr and suction irrigator. The cortex is progressively saucerized.

B. The middle fossa plate and sigmoid sinus are identified to provide early landmarks. Attention is then focused on removal of bone posterior to the sigmoid sinus.

C. The most critical step in assuring adequate exposure is the removal of bone posterior to the sigmoid sinus. Remove at least 1 cm of bone posterior to junction of the sigmoid sinus and posterior fossa dura, preferably more. Posterior fossa dura must be exposed behind the sigmoid sinus.

D. Large emissary veins are often encountered during this part of the dissection. It is best to leave these intact, if possible. Bleeding can be controlled with bone wax, surgicel, or bipolar cautery. Rarely is legation necessary.

E. It is desireable to leave a thin shell of bone over the sigmoid sinus (Bill's island). This can be removed later if it interferes with exposure. When intact Bill's island protects the sigmoid from inadvertent injury from the drill or other instrumens.

F. The sigmoid sinus is now adequately decompressed. The antrum is widely opened exposing the horizontal canal and the short process of the incus. The posterior boney external auditory canal is adequately thinned. The epitympanum is widely opened to identify the head of the malleus.

G. With the horizontal canal and incus identifying the plane of the facial nerve, bone is removed inferiorly toward the mastoid tip. This is another area that deserves adequate exposure. The digastric groove should be identified at this time.

H. As much bone as possible should be removed from the middle fossa plate. If bleeding occurs, a diamond burr will facilitate the dissection. Eventually, all bone will be removed from the middle fossa dura.

I. The sino-dural angle must be widely opened with cutting and diamond burrs. One must keep in mind the superior petrosal sinus which will run beneath the dura of the sino-dural angle. If the angle is deep, make a trough on either side with a diamond burr and remove the fragment of bone with a gimmick or blunt elevator.

J. As with the middle fossa plate, one must remove all bone over the posterior fossa plate medial to the sigmoid sinus. This disection can be facilitated by elevating the dura away from the plate with a gimmick. The suction-irrigator can then be used to retract the dura while the remaining bone is drilled away. This aids the surgeon in gauging the thickness of the bone.

K. The labyrinth should be clearly outlined by careful removal of cortical bone. The retrofacial air tract is now opened by starting posteriorly along the sigmoid sinus and posterior fossa dura and drilling medially and forward. The posterior semicircular canal has been outlined (not blue-lined) defining the superior limit of the dissection. Inferiorly, a diamond burr removes the bone over the sigmoid until the jugular bulb is clearly identified. The side of the cutting burr is used to dissect anteriorly to identify the facial nerve.

Summary: *This basic step in all oto-neurosurgical procedures has adequately decompressed the sigmoid sinus, middle fossa dura, and posterior fossa dura. The labyrinth has been clearly outlined and the vertical portion of the facial nerve positively identified. The retrofacial air tract is opened paving the way for endolymphatic sac procedures.*

2. COMPLETE SIMPLE MASTOIDECTOMY

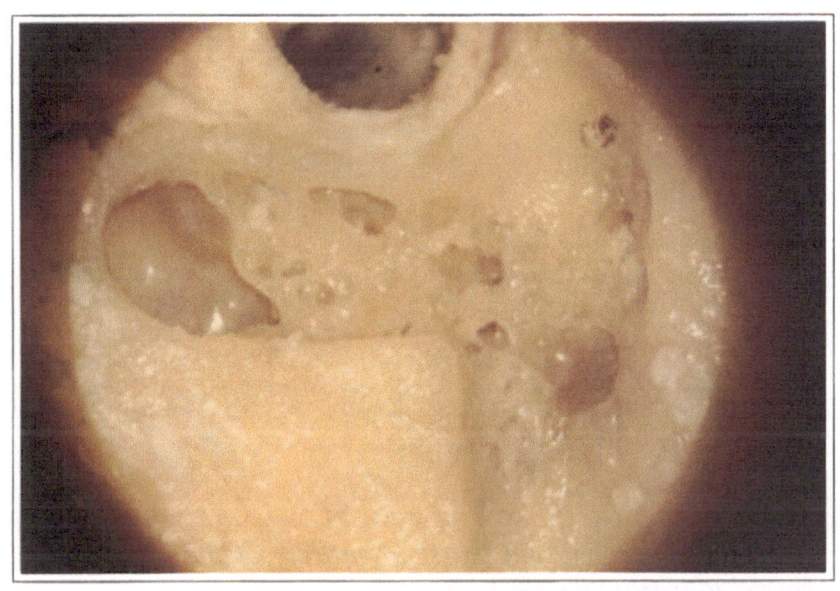

1. The dissection begins posterior to the spine of Henle.

2. The middle fossa plate and sigmoid sinus are identified to provide early landmarks. Bone posterior to the sigmoid sinus is removed to assure adequate exposure of posterior fossa dura.

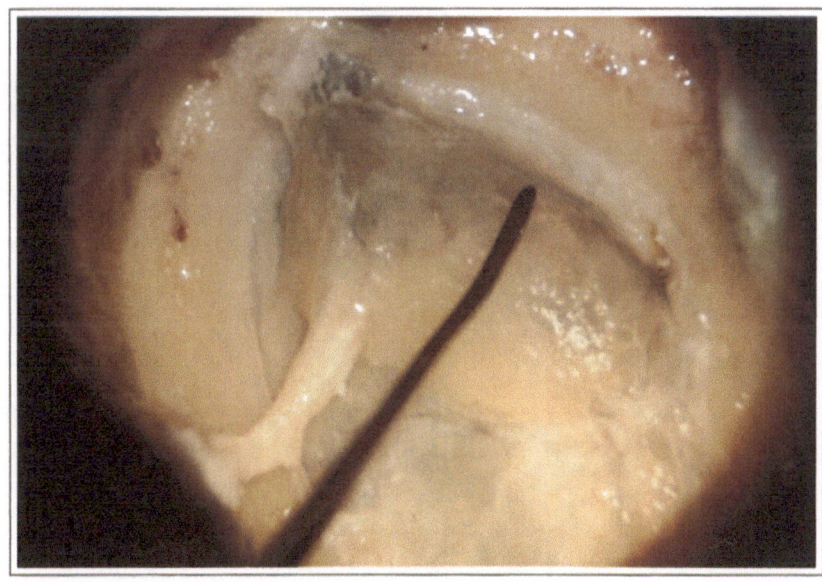

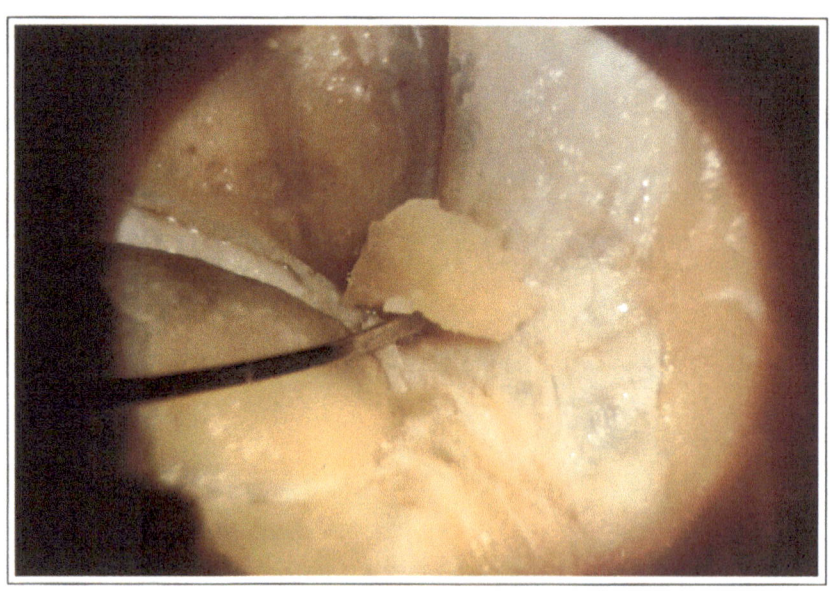

3. *The sinodural angle is widely opened.*

4. *The horizontal canal and the short process of the incus are exposed to identify the plane of the facial nerve.*

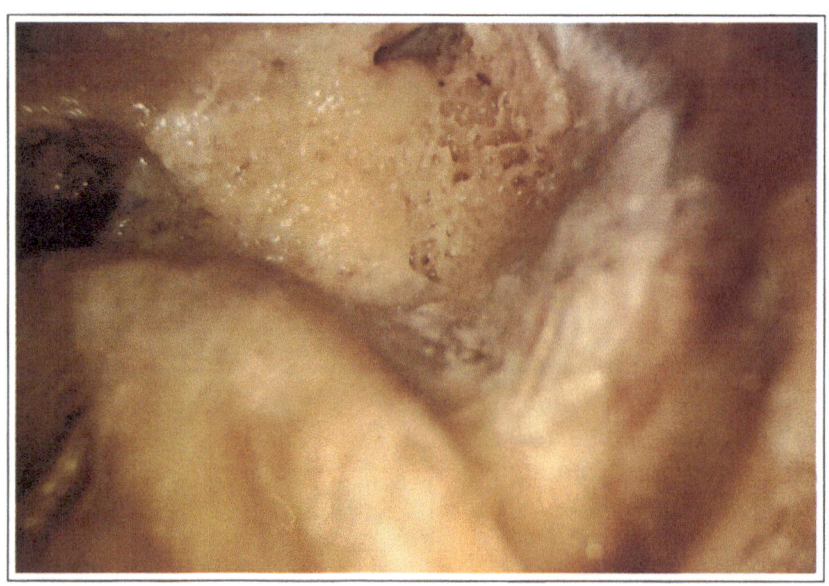

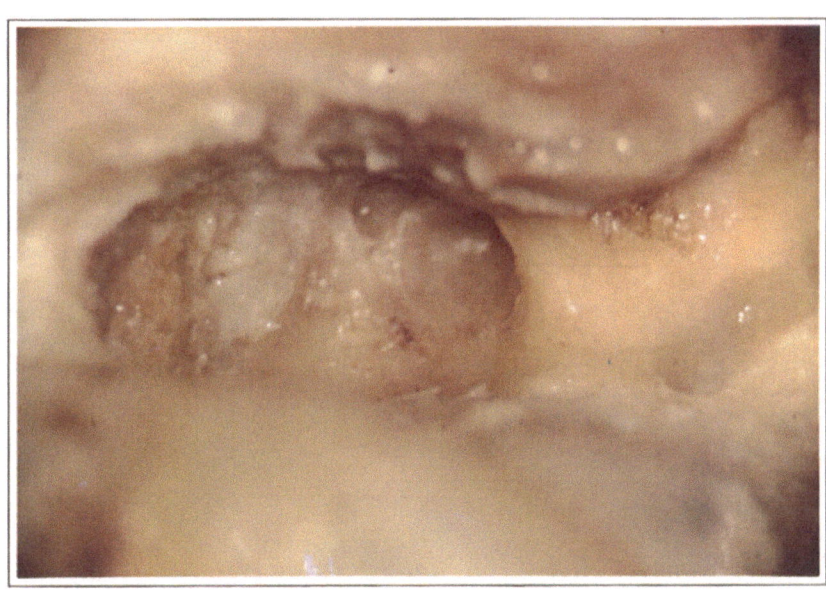

5. *The retrofacial air tract is opened, the posterior semicircular canal outlined and the jugular bulb identified.*

6. *Complete mastoidectomy has been accomplished.*

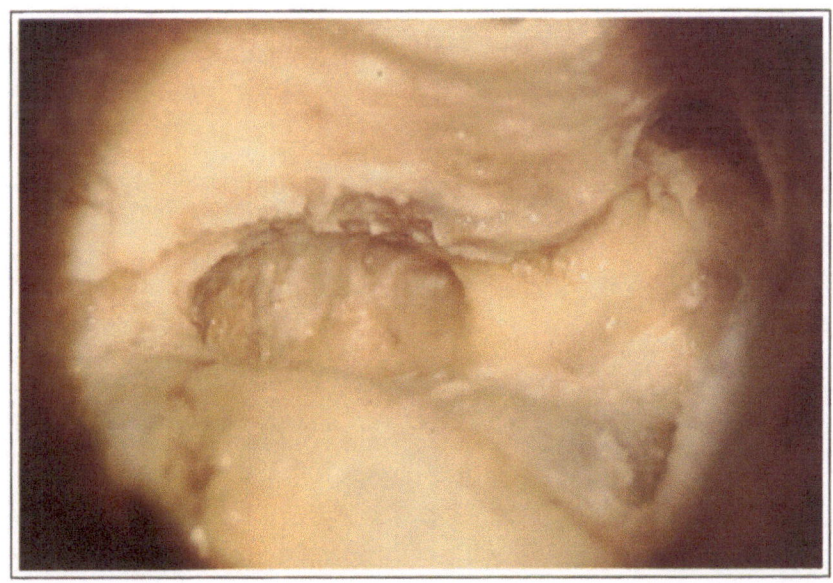

III. ENDOLYMPHATIC SAC SURGERY

This section describes the technique of identifying the endolymphatic sac, decompressing the sac, and opening the sac for shunt placement. The authors do not endorse a specific procedure for hydrops. Surgery on the endolymphatic sac requires a complete simple mastoidectomy as outlined in the preceding section.

A. A complete simple mastoidectomy has been performed. Of great importance is outlining the posterior semicircular canal to avoid inadvertent entry into this structure. The retrofacial air tract has been widely opened.

B. The sac is located by following the already decompressed sigmoid sinus and posterior fossa dura into the retrofacial air tract. This bone is removed with a diamond burr. The location of the sac is variable, but is usually identified by its texture and colour. It is usually thicker and whiter than the surrounding posterior fossa dura. Often, a prominent vessel is seen coursing over the surface of the sac.

C. Palpation of the sac usually gives a feel for the duct which passes deep to posterior canal. The limits of the dissection are the posterior fossa dura medial to the edge of the sac, the jugular bulb inferiorly, the posterior semicircular canal superiorly, and the posterior fossa dura and sigmoid sinus posteriorly. The authors favor such a wide decompression of the sac as it allows for its positive identification without jeopardizing other structures.

D. If one is to proceed with a shunt, the anterior wall is incised with a myringotomy knife or a 59S disposable beaver ophthalmic blade. The lumen is probed with a blunt instrument. The interior of the sac is quite characteristic with its glistening lumen. An endolymphatic-mastoid shunt tube can be inserted at this stage. If one prefers an endolymphatic-subarachnoid shunt, the posterior wall of the sac is opened with a fine hook until the pia-arachnoid herniates into the sac lumen. This membrane is opened and the shunt tube advanced into the subarachnoid space. This complex can then be covered with autogenous temporalis muscle.

Summary: *Wide exposure and decompression of the endolymphatic sac begins with an adequate simple mastoidectomy. By approaching the sac from posterior to anterior in the retrofacial air tract, the facial nerve is well out of harm's way, and adequate retraction of the sigmoid and posterior fossa dura is possible in case of limited exposure in a contracted mastoid.*

3. ENDOLYMPHATIC SAC DISSECTION

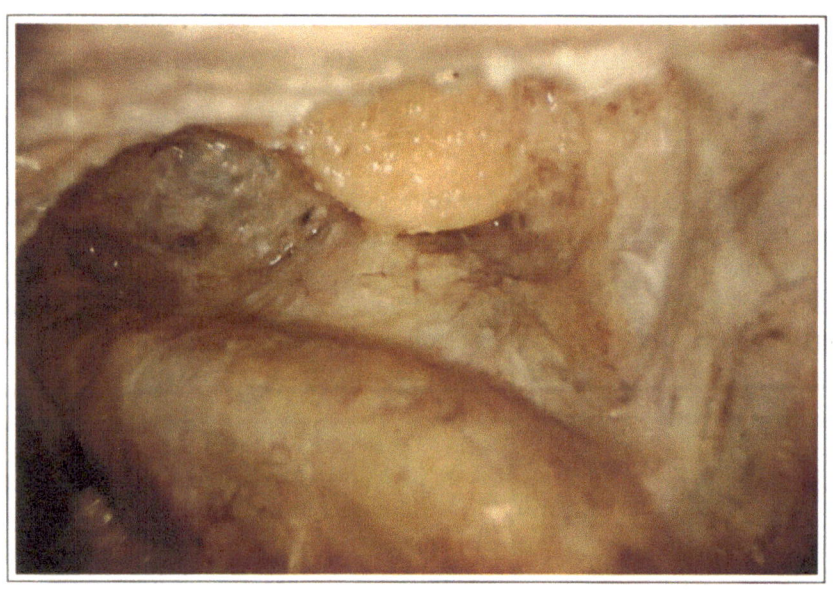

1. *A complete simple mastoidectomy has been performed outlining the posterior semicircular canal. The retrofacial air tract has been widely opened.*

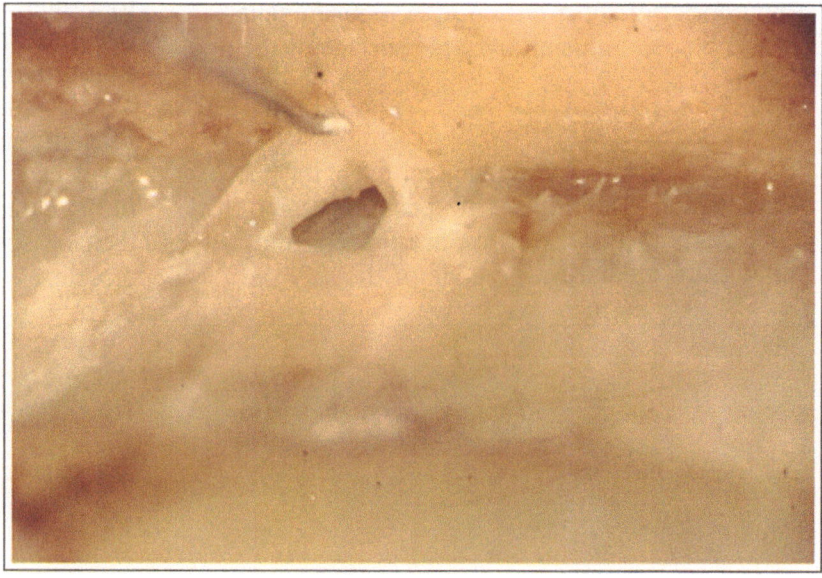

2. *The anterior wall of the sac is incised.*

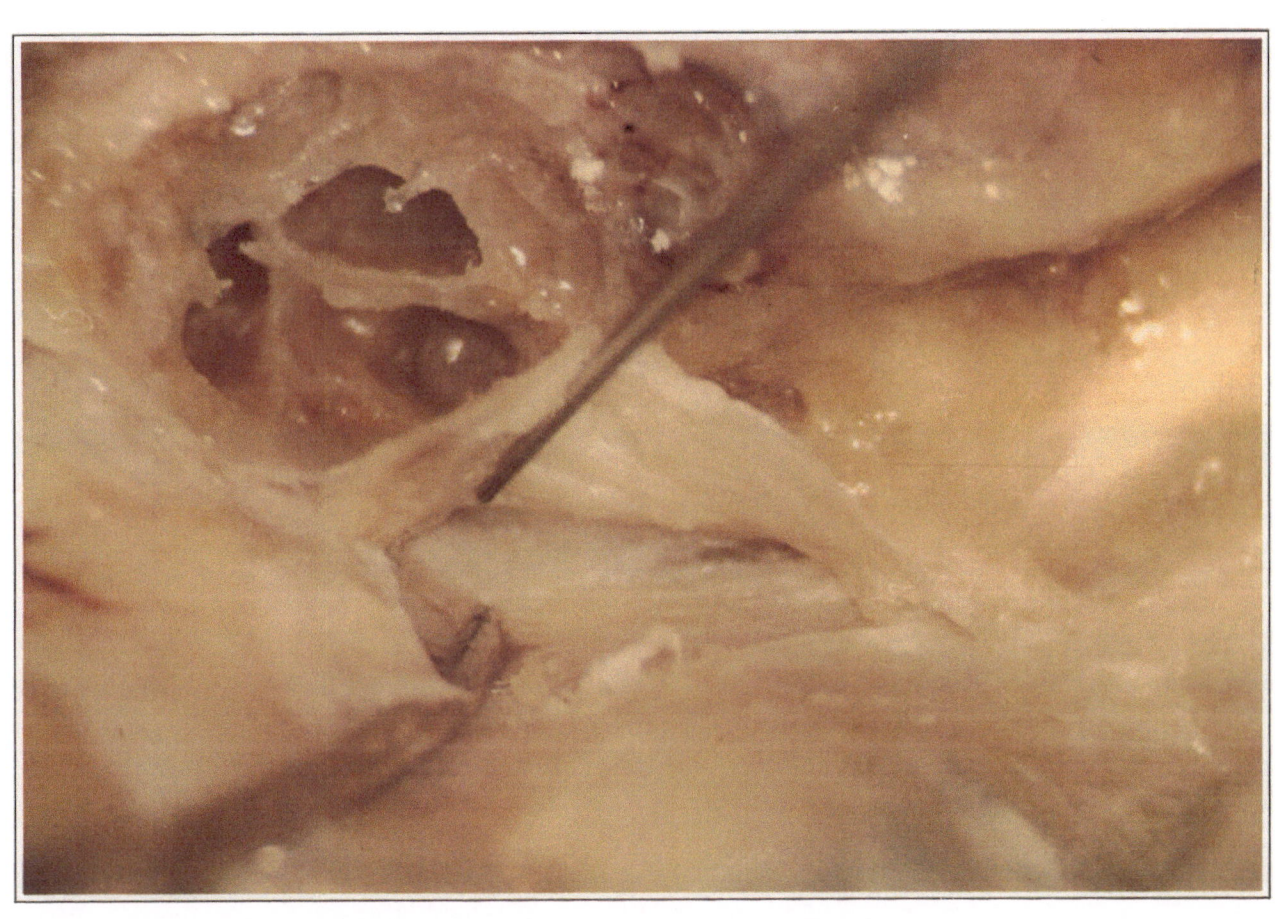

3. The sac is opened and the lumen is probed with a blunt instrument.

IV. POSTAURICULAR TRANSMASTOID LABYRINTHECTOMY

Just as the complete simple mastoidectomy provides the first building block of temporal bone surgery, the transmastoid labyrinthectomy paves the way for many oto-neurosurgical approaches to the cerebellopontine (CP) angle. This procedure must be mastered prior to attempting to expose and open the internal auditory canal (IAC).

A. A complete mastoidectomy has been accomplished as above. It is not always necessary to expose wide areas of posterior fossa and middle fossa dura when one simply wants to ablate vestibular function. In a contracted mastoid or if one plans to approach the IAC, decompression of the dural plates is important.

B. Complete removal of the boney and membranous labyrinth without compromising the facial nerve are two important goals of this approach. The dissection is initiated as far posteriorly as possible near the sino-dural angle. A cutting burr is used and the labyrinth is fenestrated. The fenestration usually occurs in the posterior canal near the common crus.

C. This fenestration is enlarged superiorly and inferiorly until the orientation of the superior and posterior canals are clearly seen. The superior canal lies at a relatively deep level this far posteriorly. As one progresses anteriorly toward the ampulla of the superior canal, the plane of dissection becomes more superficial.

D. The cutting burr then dissects anteriorly toward the horizontal canal. The horizontal canal is fenestrated with the side of the cutting burr. This is important as it provides for more efficient dissection utilizing the flutes of the burr, and also leaves a shell of bone to protect the facial nerve.

E. With the side of the burr, the horizontal canal is removed superiorly to inferiorly in the direction of the facial nerve. The ampullated end of the posterior canal is removed when the facial nerve has been identified in this fashion, as the ampulla may actually be beneath the facial.

F. If any of the membranous superior canal remains, it is removed at this time. Bleeding from the subarcuate artery is common and is usually easily controlled with a diamond burr, or, in rare cases, the bipolar cautery.

G. With the semicircular canal exenterated, one should now have a clear view of the vestibule with its membranous structures, the maculae of the utricle and saccule. Bone is removed beneath the facial in order to adequately expose the vestibule. The contents of the vestibule are easily aspirated or removed with an instrument. Caution should be used when drilling in or near the vestibule as its medial wall represents the lateral end of the IAC. Opening the medial wall of the vestibule could result in potential damage to the facial nerve and cerebrospinal fluid (CSF) leakage.

H. With the labyrinth removed, one should be able to see the course of the endolymphatic duct which appears as a white thread-like structure exiting inferiorly from the vestibule and heading for the sac. The ampulla of the superior canal often reveals a white dot (Mike's white dot) medial to it representing the end of the superior vestibular nerve, a very important landmark in translabyrinthine surgery.

Summary: *The labyrinth is systematically removed by starting the dissection posteriorly where there are no important structures to jeopardize. The facial nerve is found by removing the horizontal canal with the side of the burr leaving a thin shell of bone to protect the facial. The semicircular canals provide a roadmap to the vestibule. The contents of the vestibule and all remaining neuroepithelium are meticulously removed. This procedure opens the door for the translabyrinthine approach to the CP angle.*

V. TRANSLABYRINTHINE INTERNAL AUDITORY CANAL EXPOSURE

Having accomplished a complete mastoidectomy and transmastoid labyrinthectomy, the next oto-neurosurgical building block is exposure of the internal auditory canal (IAC). This will provide access to the cerebellopontine (CP) angle. The authors prefer to skeletonize the IAC after the posterior and middle fossa plates have been removed as described above. This enhances exposure by allowing retraction of the dura.

A. Critical to translabyrinthine surgery is positive identification of the facial nerve. The mastoid segment of the facial nerve is skeletonized by drilling forward in the retrofacial air tract until the pink streak of the facial is seen. A diamond burr and copious irrigation are then used to follow the nerve superiorly toward the epitympanum. Removal of this ledge of bone over the facial gives additional exposure to the lateral end of the IAC. Often the stapedius muscle is seen and may be confused with the facial. It courses medial to the facial and lateral to the vestibule. It may cause some nuisance bleeding that is best managed by watchful waiting. The epitympanum must be widely opened to provide visualization of the incudo-malleal articulation and the cochleariform process.

B. Prior to bone removal over the IAC, the surgeon fixes in his mind's eye the orientation of the IAC. It lies between the ampullae of the superior and posterior semicircular canals coursing inferiorly and medially toward the porus acousticus. The canal lies in a much deeper plane posteriorly with a thick plate of bone over the porus. Looking at the temporal bone from behind will assist in understanding the orientation of the IAC. Appreciating the varying thickness of bone over the IAC from vestibule to porus greatly facilitates dissection.

C. Dissection begins superiorly to the IAC with a cutting burr. A trough is created above the IAC, and subsequently below the IAC until at least 270 degrees of bone have been removed from around the canal. A tract of pneumatization is often found superior to the canal, aiding in dissection. A thin shell of bone is left on the IAC to protect its contents. Inferiorly, the dissection proceeds in a similar fashion. The jugular bulb is skeletonized and marks the inferior limit of bone removal. A trough is created between the IAC and jugular bulb until one is well around the inferior portion of the IAC. Again, a thin layer of bone is left on the canal.

D. Prior to drilling away the thick bone over the porus, the posterior fossa dura is elevated away from the porus acousticus. The bone is thinned with a cutting burr.

E. The final dissection of the IAC utilizes a diamond burr to thin the bone down to the level of the dura superiorly and inferiorly in the troughs created above and below the IAC. These paths are united laterally by careful removal of bone at the lateral end of the IAC. This brings into view the transverse crest. By gently manipulating the remaining cap of bone over the IAC with a gimmick, a saddle-shaped piece of bone should be able to be removed bringing into full view the dural-covered IAC contents. Removing the porus in this fashion in one piece avoids tedious and dangerous drilling over the IAC.

F. Although well around the IAC, often at this stage there will still be a wedge of bone superiorly and inferiorly. This can be removed by gently retracting the contents of the IAC with the suction-irrigator and drilling forward onto these "points" with a diamond drill.

G. One structure that deserves attention now is the cochlear aqueduct. One should make a diligent search for this structure as one drills inferior to the IAC. Coursing between the jugular bulb and the inferior border of the IAC, the cochlear aqueduct delineates the anterior limit of dissection. Dissecting anteriorly and medial to this structure places cranial nerves IX, X and XI in jeopardy. CSF will often emanate from the cochlear aqueduct when it is opened.

H. The only task remaining prior to opening the dura is identification of the facial nerve as it enters the IAC. If enough bone has been removed superiorly to the IAC at its lateral end, Bill's bar is often quite obvious. If not, continue drilling forward with a diamond burr (making sure that the drill is rotating away from the facial) until the labyrinthine segment of the facial nerve is seen.

I. Exposure is now adequate for gaining access to the cerebellopontine (CP) angle. Prior to violating the subarachnoid space, the surgical field should be irrigated with an antibiotic-containing solution and fresh drapes placed about the wound. The dura is opened at the lateral end of the IAC immediately over the superior vestibular nerve (SVN) with a sharp right angle hook. The same hook palpates Bill's bar deep to the SVN and then gently lifts the SVN away from the facial. The facial nerve should now be visualized as one retracts the SVN. A blunt right angle hook now develops the plane between the SVN (or tumor) and the facial.

Summary: *Translabyrinthine exposure of the IAC paves the way for removal of CP angle lesions, section of vestibular and cochlear nerves, and total decompression of the facial nerve. If bone removal has been performed satisfactorily, this approach provides adequate access for total removal of posterior fossa lesions.*

4. TRANSLABYRINTHINE DISSECTION

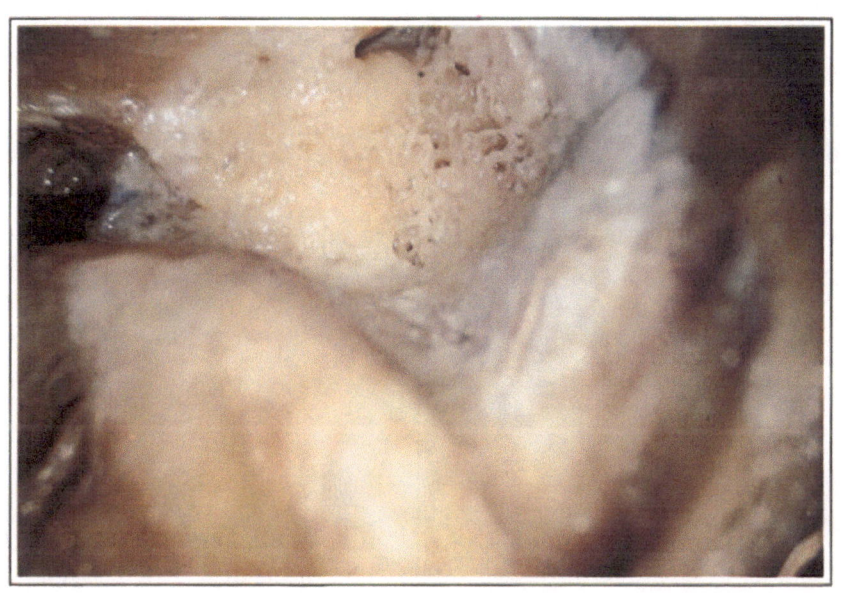

1. *A complete simple mastoidectomy has been performed. The middle and posterior fossa plate are thinned and the sino-dural angle is completely opened to provide adequate exposure of the vestibule.*

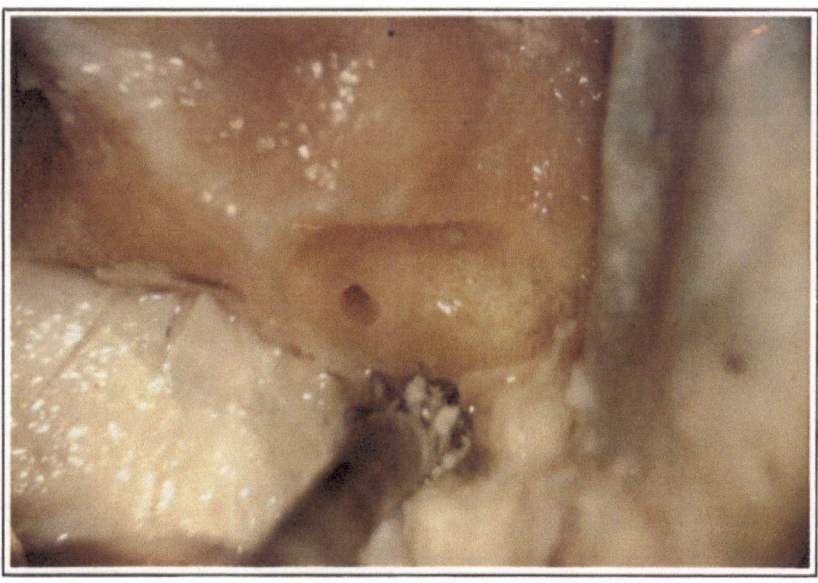

2. *The dissection is initiated posteriorly near the sino-dural angle.*

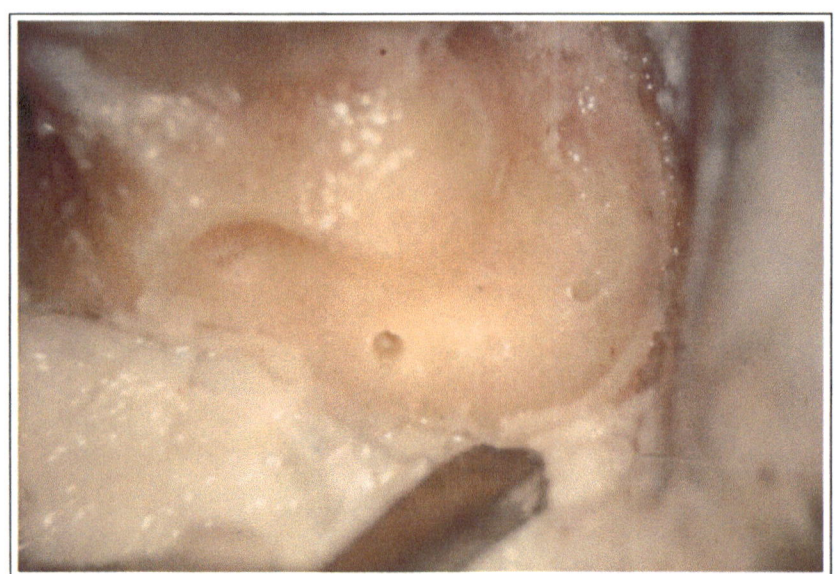

3. *The fenestration is enlarged superiorly and inferiorly.*

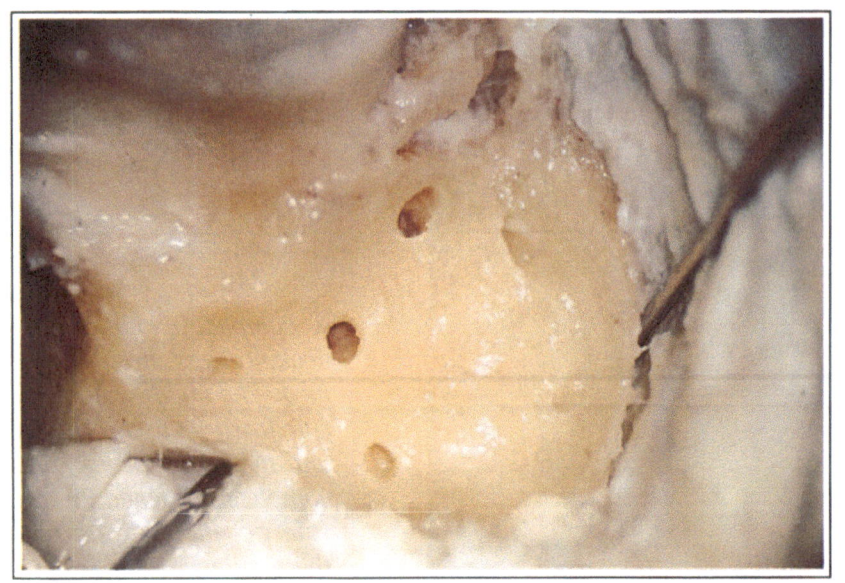

4. *Semicircular canals are fenestrated.*

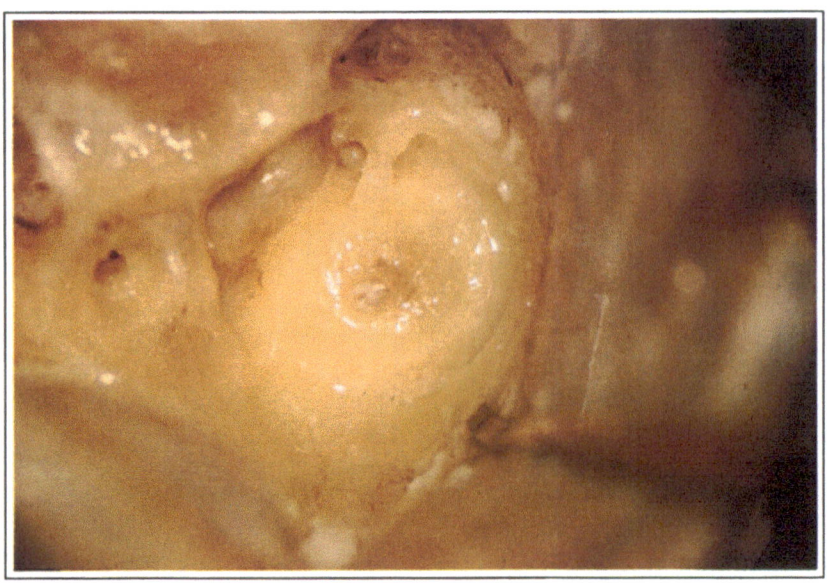

5. *The vestibule is opened and the subarcuate artery identified.*

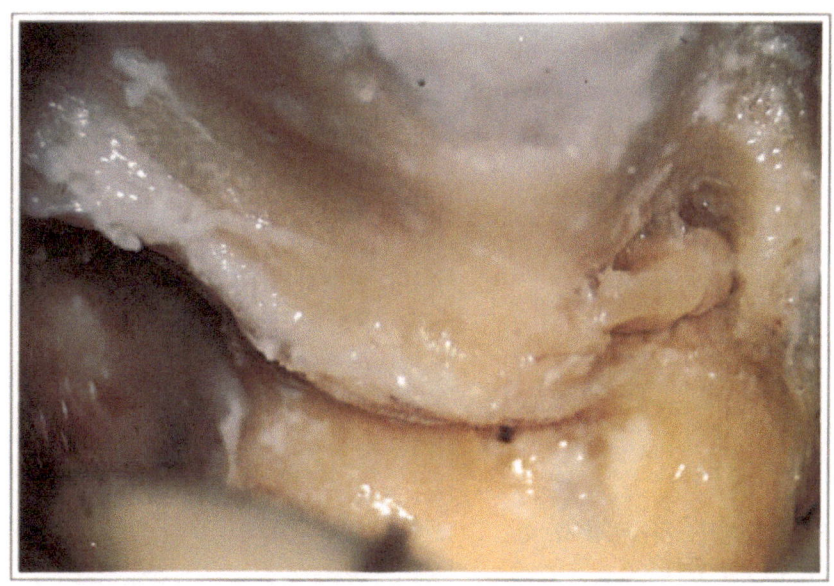

6. *Horizontal and tympanic facial nerve are skeletonized and the bone is removed over the lateral end of the IAC.*

7. *Bone is removed over the middle and posterior fossa dura and drilling is continued over the porus acousticus.*

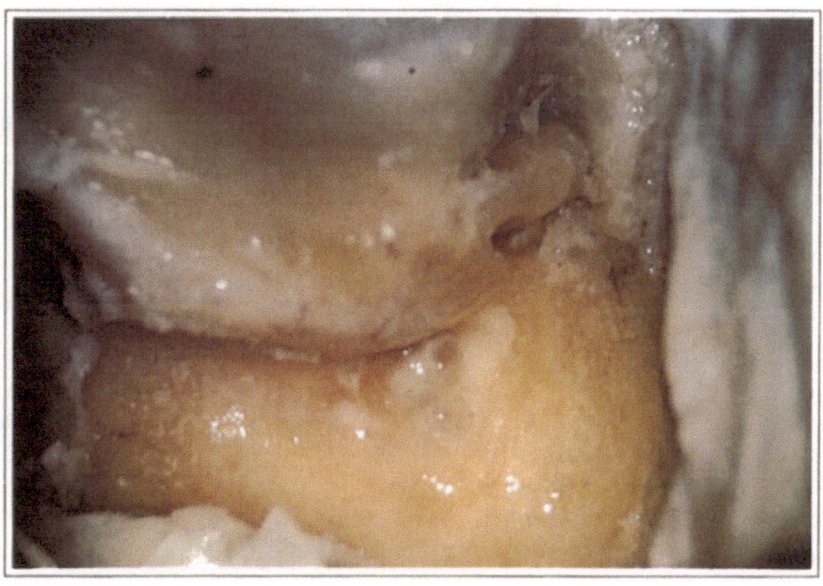

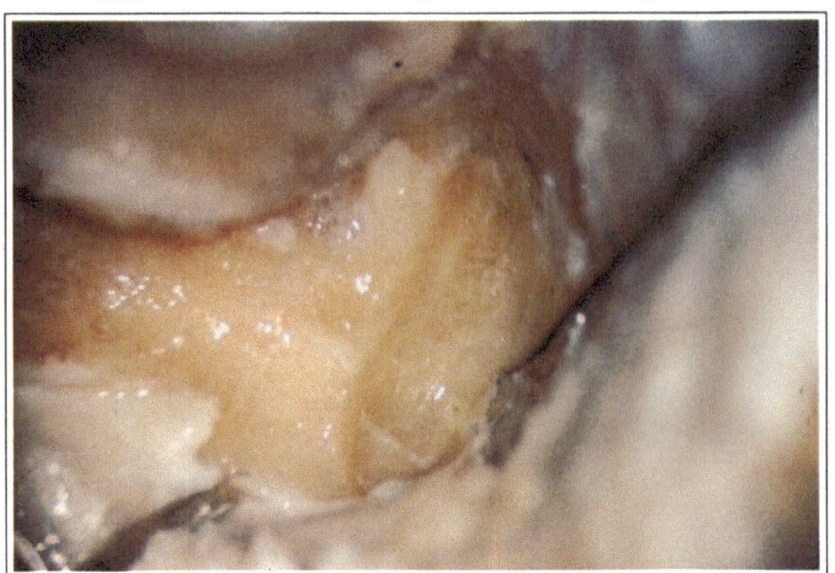

8. *A trough is created superior to the IAC.*

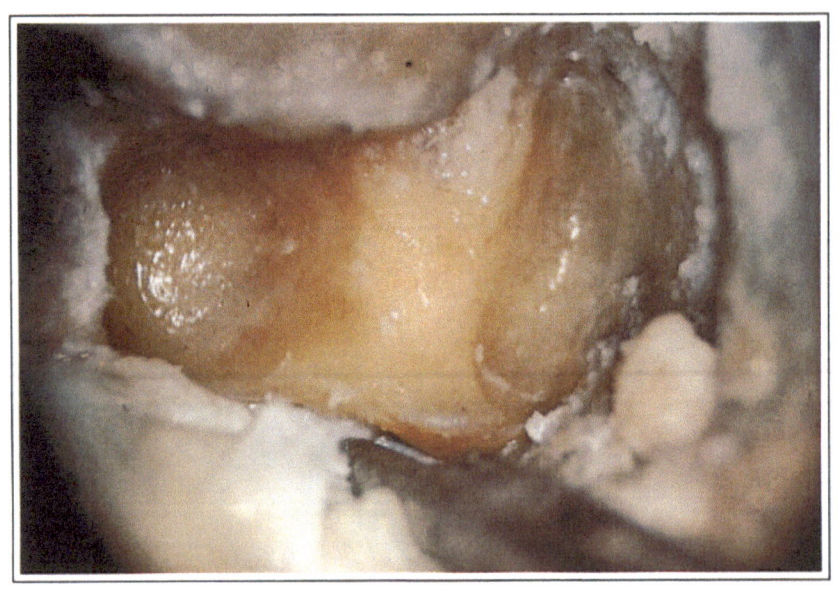

9. *A second trough is drilled inferior to the IAC to expose at least 270 degrees around the IAC.*

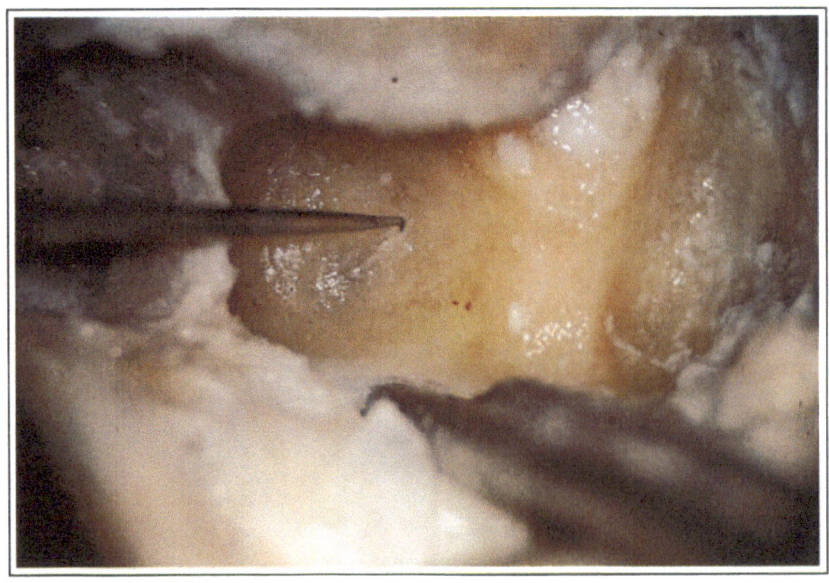

10. *The instrument demonstrates the cochlear aqueduct.*

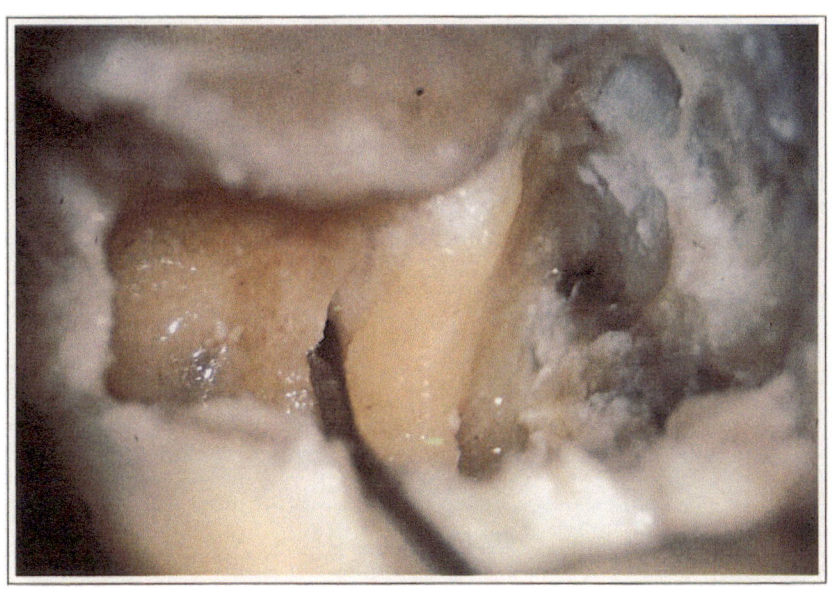

11. The bone over the porus is dissected from the dura of the IAC.

12. The entire porus is removed en bloc.

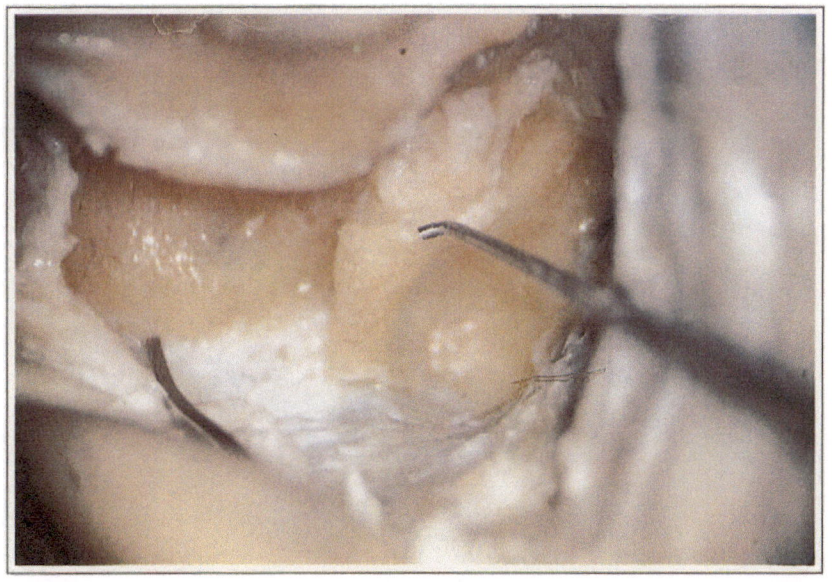

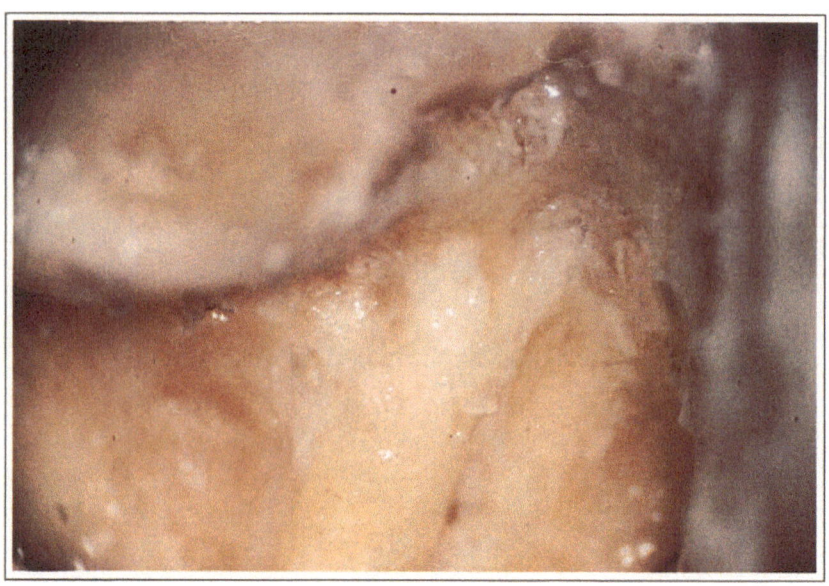

13. The dura over the IAC is exposed.

14. The instrument indicates Bill's Bar.

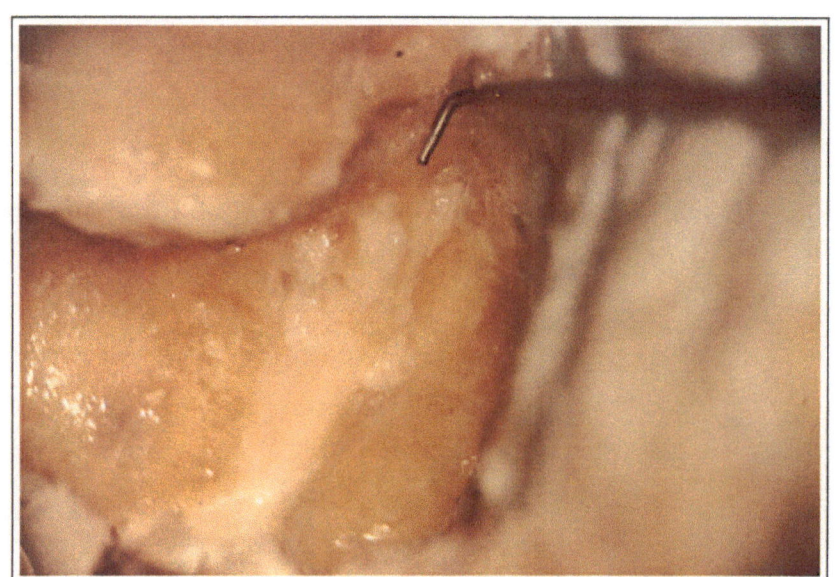

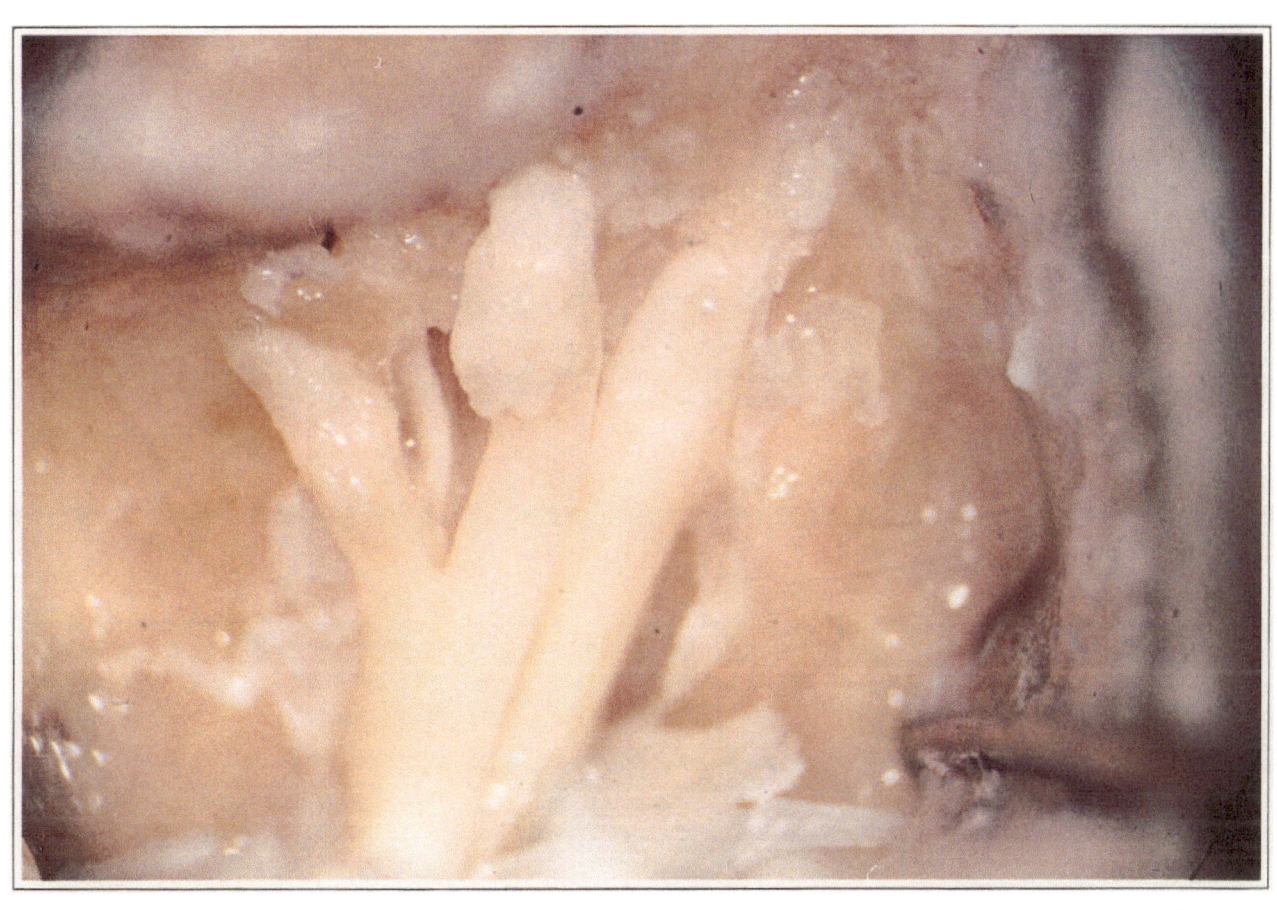

15. *With the dura of the IAC opened, the facial, superior vestibular, inferior vestibular and singular nerves are seen.*

VI. TRANSLABYRINTHINE REMOVAL OF ACOUSTIC TUMORS

Having adequately exposed the contents of the IAC, a brief discussion regarding the technical aspects of acoustic tumor dissection is in order.

A. The surgeon must first be absolutely certain of the location of the facial nerve. The greatest single advantage of the translabyrinthine approach to acoustic tumor removal is positive identification of the facial nerve prior to tumor removal. The plane between the facial and tumor must be developed at the lateral end of the IAC. This plane of dissection is continued posteriorly toward the porus. The inferior vestibular nerve is now removed with a sharp hook and reflected posteriorly. It is critical now to explore the end of the IAC with a blunt hook to make certain that no tumor has been left in the canal.

B. The dura will now be opened over the posterior fossa portion of the tumor. With Jacobson scissors, a dural flap is created, cutting along the superior petrosal sinus superiorly and inferiorly along the sigmoid sinus and jugular bulb. These cuts are united at the porus, basing the flap posteriorly. The flap is grasped with a bayonet forceps and insinuated over the tumor capsule toward the brainstem. This maneuver actually begins the development of the plane between the tumor and the brainstem. A flow of CSF is obtained, thereby decompressing the posterior fossa, by blunt dissection inferior to the tumor. Opening the arachnoid between the inferior pole of the tumor and the jugular bulb usually results in brisk egress of CSF.

C. Two structures must be kept in mind while opening the dura: the petrosal vein and the anterior inferior cerebellar artery (AICA). The petrosal vein is located superiorly and can bleed profusely if disrupted. AICA is usually located inferior to large tumors, but can be found almost anywhere in the CP angle. Heeding these two structures, and with adequate exposure of the tumor, one first biopsies the lesion for histologic confirmation. Extensive gutting of the tumor is performed by morselizing the tumor with forceps and using the House-Urban rotary suction-dissector to debulk the tumor. As the tumor is gutted, it will collapse upon itself making dissection of the capsule easier.

D. When dissecting the capsule away from the brainstem and cerebellum it is important to stay within the relatively avascular plane between the arachnoid and the tumor capsule. Continue rolling the gutted tumor away from the facial. Dissection is always most difficult at the porus and it is here where the facial is likely to be injured. Positive identification of the facial at the porus is critical in order to minimize the chance for injury.

E. The facial is relocated at the end of the IAC and traced toward the porus. The tumor remaining at the porus is removed by staying within the plane of the facial and the tumor with a blunt hook. This dissection is tedious but well worth the effort to preserve facial nerve function. The remaining piece of tumor is dissected free and removed.

F. With total tumor removal accomplished, the wound is irrigated with an antibiotic-containing solution. Usually there is some bleeding in the tumor bed from feeder vessels. These are easily controlled with bipolar cautery. Oozing from around large vessels or nerves is best controlled with pledgets of microfibrillar collagen. With hemostasis complete, the size of the defect is assessed. If a large cavern remains, as would be the case following removal of a large tumor, strips of gelfoam soaked in saline are placed in the tumor bed. This helps to obliterate dead space and discourages the development of a hematoma. Surgicel is not used as its swelling is unpredictable and could result in brainstem compromise.

G. Closure is accomplished by obtaining abdominal fat, cutting the fat into thin strips, and insinuating the fat into the dural defect. The fat should be packed tightly, but should not be allowed to prolapse into the CP angle. The wound is closed in layers with absorbable suture.

Summary: *Adequate exposure through meticulous temporal bone dissection is the first critical step in acoustic tumor removal. This allows positive identification of the facial nerve. Tumor removal is accomplished by gutting the tumor and removal piecemeal. Always, the surgeon must respect the complicated and crucial vascular anatomy of the CP angle.*

VII. RETROLABYRINTHINE SURGERY

The retrolabyrinthine approach of the CP angle allows the surgeon to manage various posterior fossa conditions without violating the labyrinth, thus destroying hearing. The principal use of this approach is to section the vestibular nerve for vertigo. It can also be used for performing vascular decompression surgery, although the retrosigmoid approach is more versatile for these procedures.

A. The surgery begins with a complete mastoidectomy and identification of the endolymphatic sac. It is imperative that the surgeon remove at least 2 cm of bone posterior to the sigmoid sinus.

B. At this time the surgeon instructs the anesthesiologist to administer 250 cc of 20% mannitol by slow intravenous infusion. This is followed by 40 mg of lasix given intravenously. These agents greatly facilitate exposure by dehydrating the brain.

C. The orientation of the semicircular canals should be clearly in mind and the posterior canal should be outlined. The surgeon needs to remove as much bone as possible between the posterior canal and posterior fossa dura without fenestrating the canal.

D. Complete decompression of the middle and posterior fossa plates is carried out. The sinodural angle is drilled out down to the dura over the superior petrosal sinus.

E. Inferiorly, the dissection is carried down to the jugular bulb. The retrofacial air tract should be widely opened.

F. The wound is irrigated with an antibiotic-containing solution prior to opening the dura. An anteriorly-based dural flap is created by opening the dura superiorly along the superior petrosal sinus, inferiorly above the jugular bulb, and uniting these incisions by cutting just medial to the sigmoid sinus and lateral to the endolymphatic sac. The pia-arachnoid herniates into the subdural space and can be opened with a sharp hook, allowing a brisk flow of CSF.

G. One may wish to place a suture in the dural flap to provide forward retraction. A moist cottonoid is placed over the cerebellum, which is gently compressed. Gentle retraction of the cerebellum gives adequate exposure to the CP angle. The eighth nerve complex is found by following an imaginary line posteriorly from the horizontal canal. A branch of the petrosal vein may be seen near the root entry zone of the eighth nerve. AICA is generally medial to the eighth nerve complex.

H. Viewing the eighth nerve under 10x or 16x usually shows a difference in coloration between the vestibular (superior) and cochlear (inferior) portions of the nerve. A vessel often accompanies the cleavage plane. The vestibular portion is sectioned by first cutting into the superior aspect of the nerve with a scissors, and then gently feathering through the fibers with a sharp hook. When a complete section has been achieved, the cut ends of the nerve usually spring apart. One must keep in mind the facial nerve which lies deep to the eighth nerve, and AICA which often lies between seven and eight.

I. Having sectioned the vestibular nerve, closure is accomplished with strips of fat just as in acoustic tumor surgery. The CP angle is inspected for other signs of pathology prior to closing.

Summary: *The retrolabyrinthine approach is best suited for sectioning the vestibular nerve. Mandatory to this approach is adequate exposure far posterior to the sigmoid sinus. For approaching the fifth cranial nerve or lower cranial nerves, the authors prefer the retrosigmoid approach described below.*

5. RETROLABYRINTHINE APPROACH (VESTIBULAR NERVE SECTION)

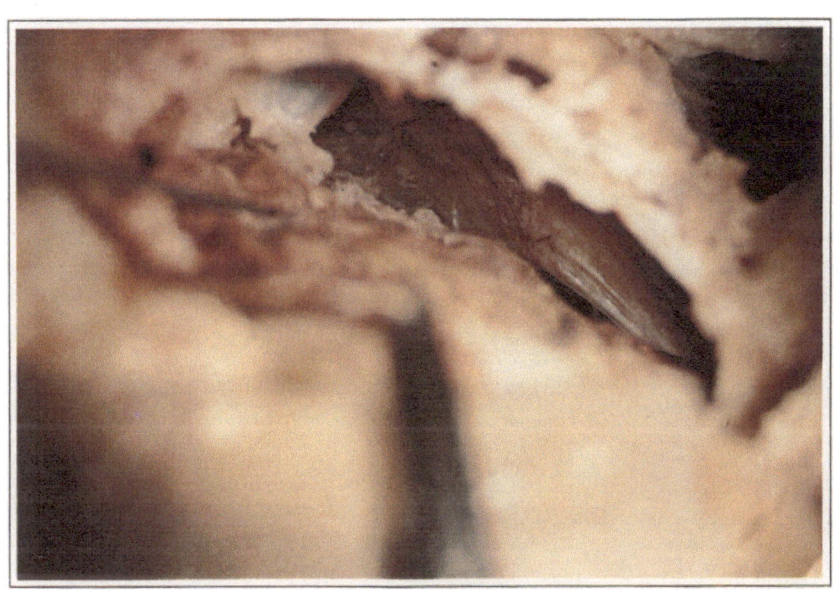

1. *Following adequate bone removal, the dura is opened between the sigmoid sinus and posterior semicircular canal.*

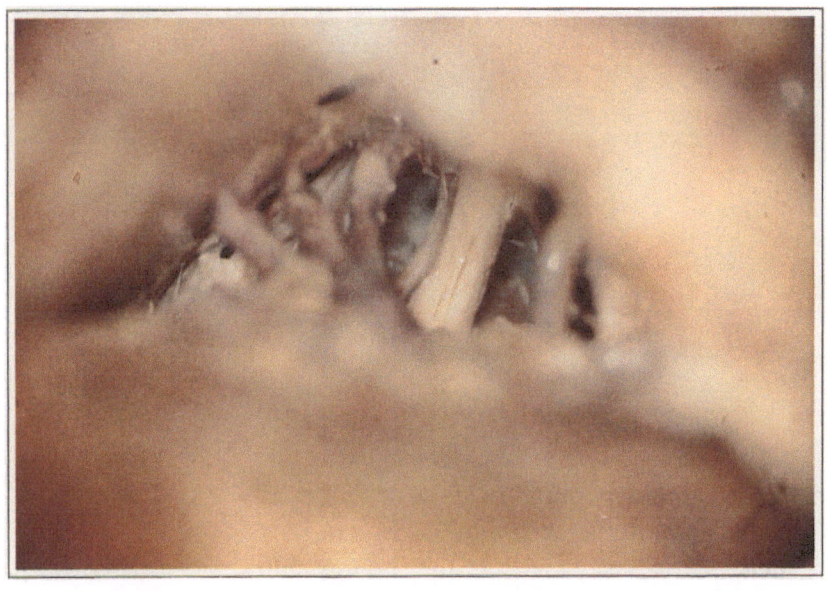

2. *Gentle retraction of the cerebellum demonstrates the eighth nerve complex in the cerebellopontine angle.*

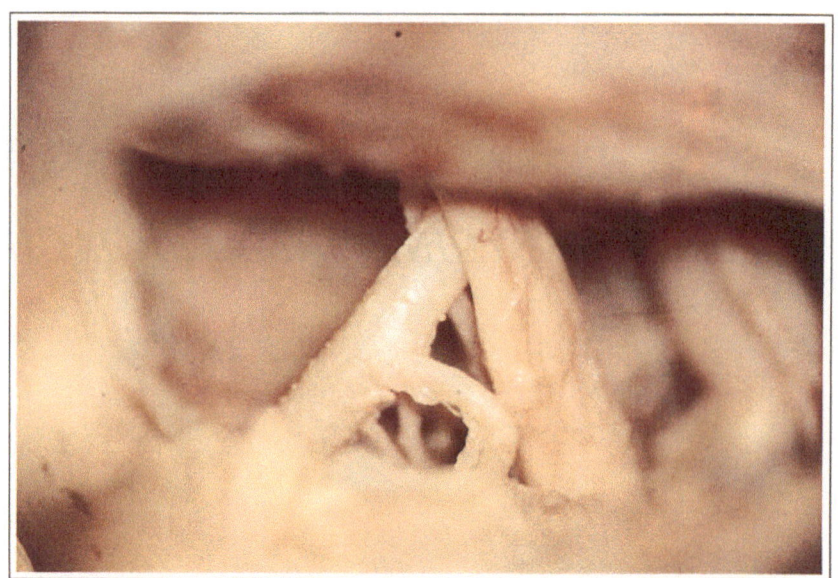

3. *The eighth nerve is well visualized with a large loop of AICA between VII and VIII.*

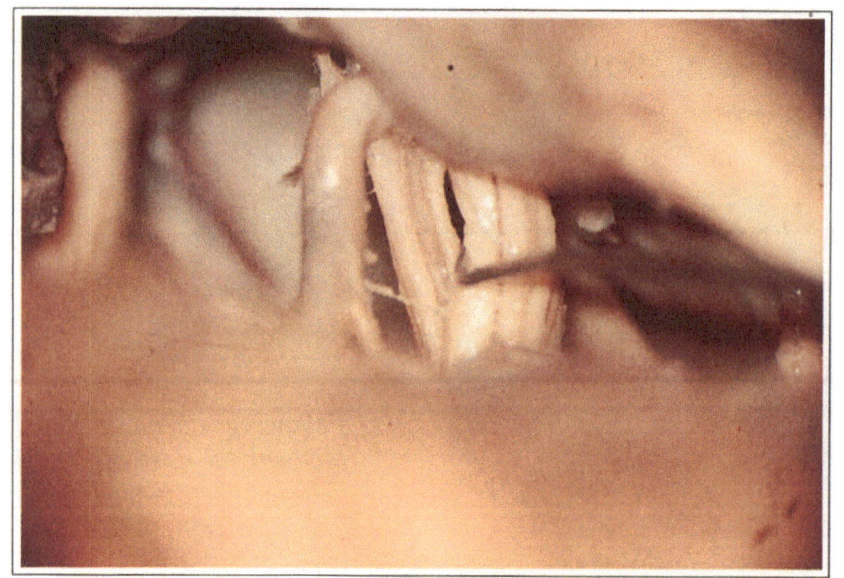

4. *Retraction of the eighth nerve reveals the facial nerve.*

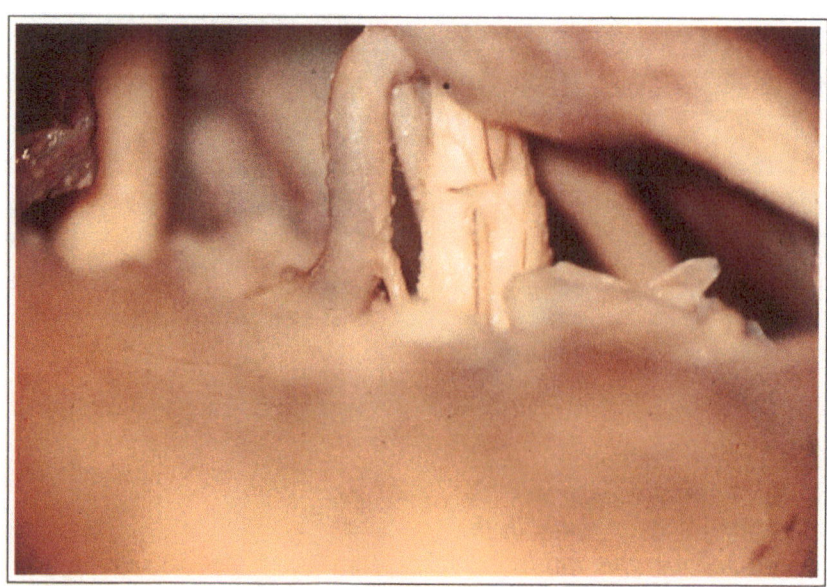

5. *The vestibular portion of the eighth nerve is sectioned.*

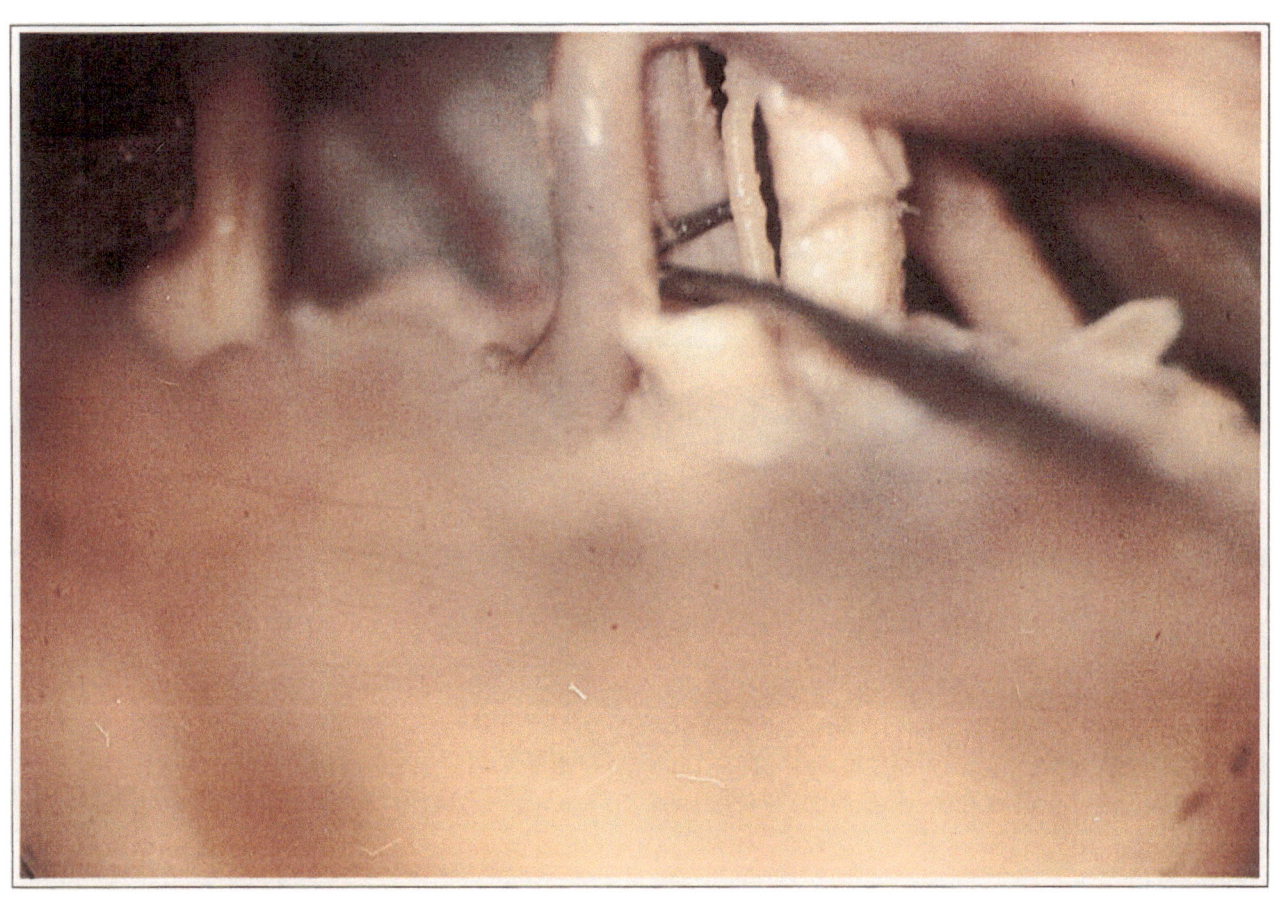

6. *The nervus intermedius and facial nerve are seen following adequate vestibular neurectomy.*

VIII. RETROSIGMOID SURGERY

Because it affords wider exposure to the posterior fossa and CP angle, the retrosigmoid approach is preferred for vascular decompression procedures on the V, VII, VIII, IX, X and XI cranial nerves.One must bear in mind that it requires more cerebellar retraction and hence has more inherent morbidity.

A. The skin incision is described in the first section. Like the retrolabyrinth approach, it must be well posterior.The incision is carried down into the neck for a distance of roughly 3 cm below the mastoid tip.

B. The dissection is identical as for the retrolabyrinthine approach, including the administration of mannitol and lasix.

C. Once adequate retrolabyrinthine bone removal has been accomplished, a large rongeur is used to remove an additional 3-4 cm of bone from the subocciput behind the sigmoid. A large section of posterior fossa dura is hence exposed behind the sigmoid.

D. The wound is irrigated prior to creating a posteriorly-based dural flap. The dura is opened along the posterior margin of the sigmoid, with posterior limbs being made at both ends of the cut. The arachnoid is opened and CSF allowed to escape.

E. A cottonoid protects the cerebellar hemisphere, which is gently compressed. If necessary, traction sutures can be placed to retract the sigmoid anteriorly. The CP angle can be visualized by retracting the cerebellum posteriorly.

F. Generally, this approach provides more working room than the retrolabyrinthine approach when one desires to decompress vascular loops from the V, VII and VIII cranial nerves. More room is generated inferiorly and superiorly, allowing safer and more facile work on the lower cranial nerves.

G. The authors use shredded teflon felt to cushion the cranial nerve from the vascular loop, once it has been identified.

H. Closure is accomplished by a watertight dural suture line, and strips of fat placed into the mastoid and over the suture line.

Summary: *Retrosigmoid surgery is a logical extention of retrolabyrinthine surgery, made possible by additional removal of bone posterior to the sigmoid and extending the skin incision into the upper neck. As more cerebellar retraction is necessary with this approach, one must be aware of the increased potential for morbidity.*

6. RETROSIGMOID APPROACH

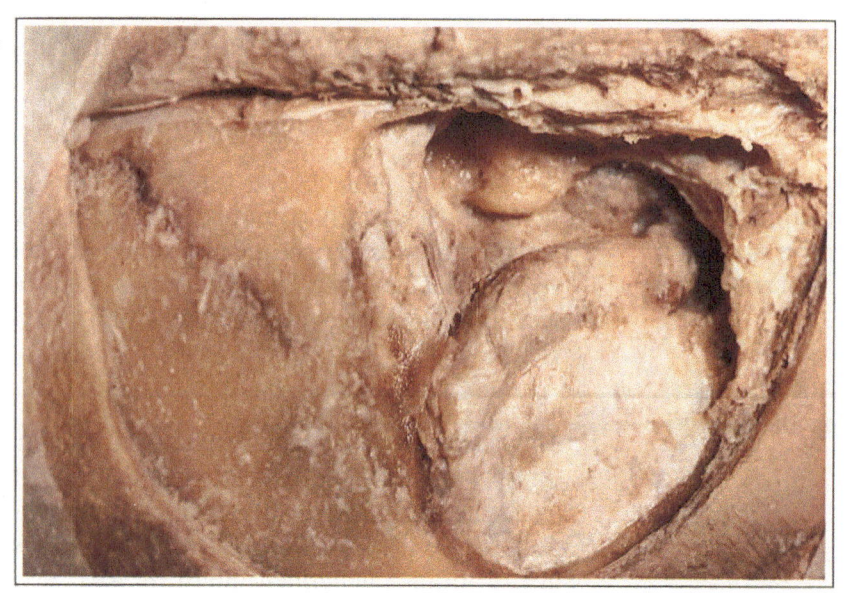

1. *Adequate bone removal far behind the sigmoid sinus and demonstrating the labyrinth.*

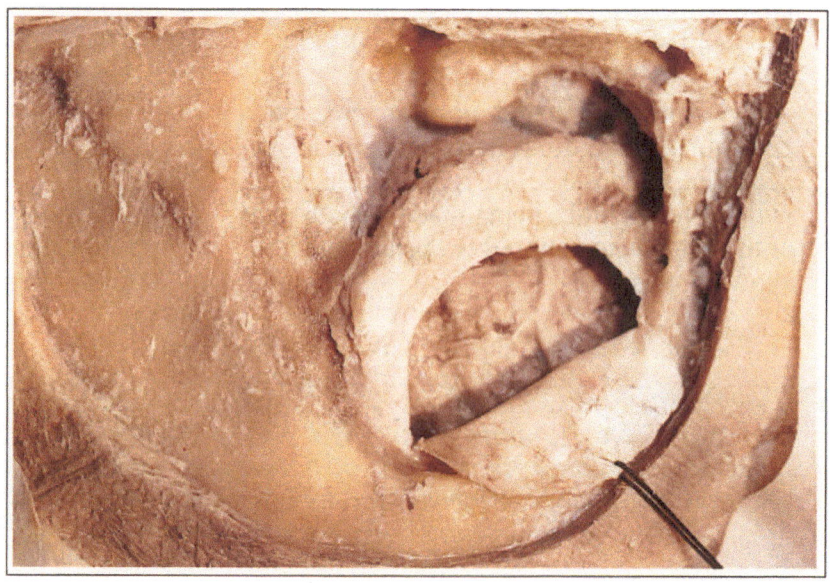

2. *The dura is opened behind the sigmoid sinus.*

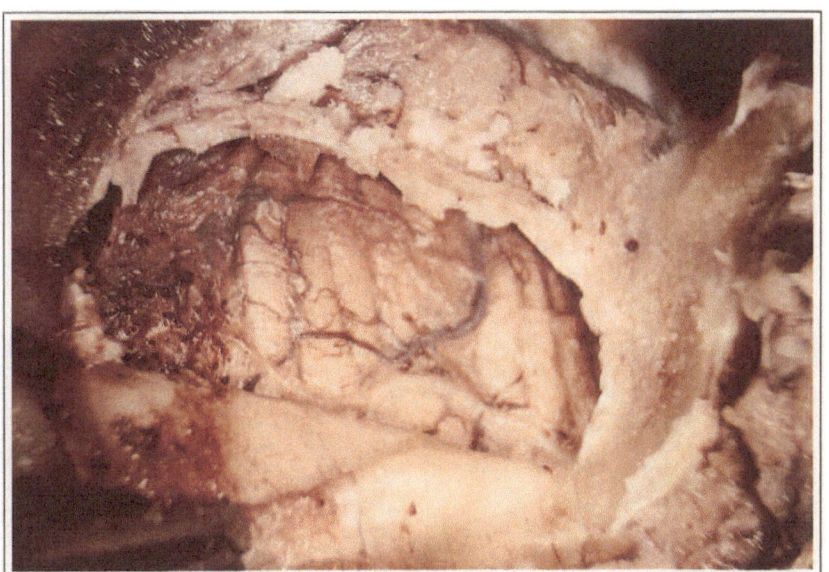

3. *The cerebellum is seen and gently retracted.*

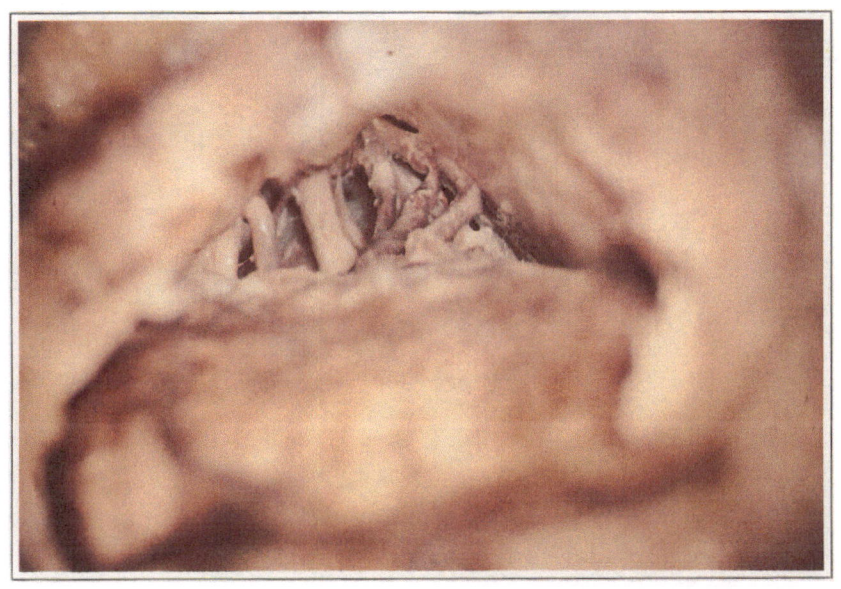

4. *The cerebellopontine angle exposed through the retro-sigmoid approach.*

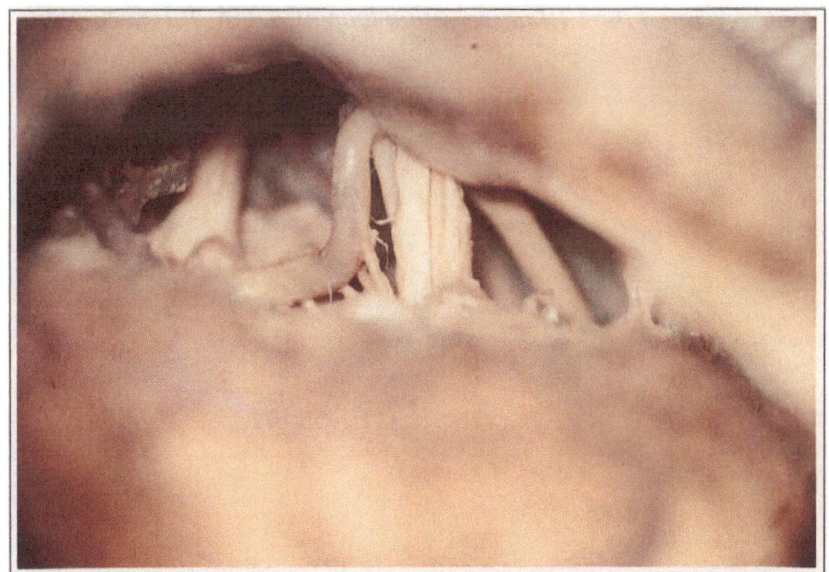

5. *The V nerve seen at the far left and the VIII nerve in the center of the field.*

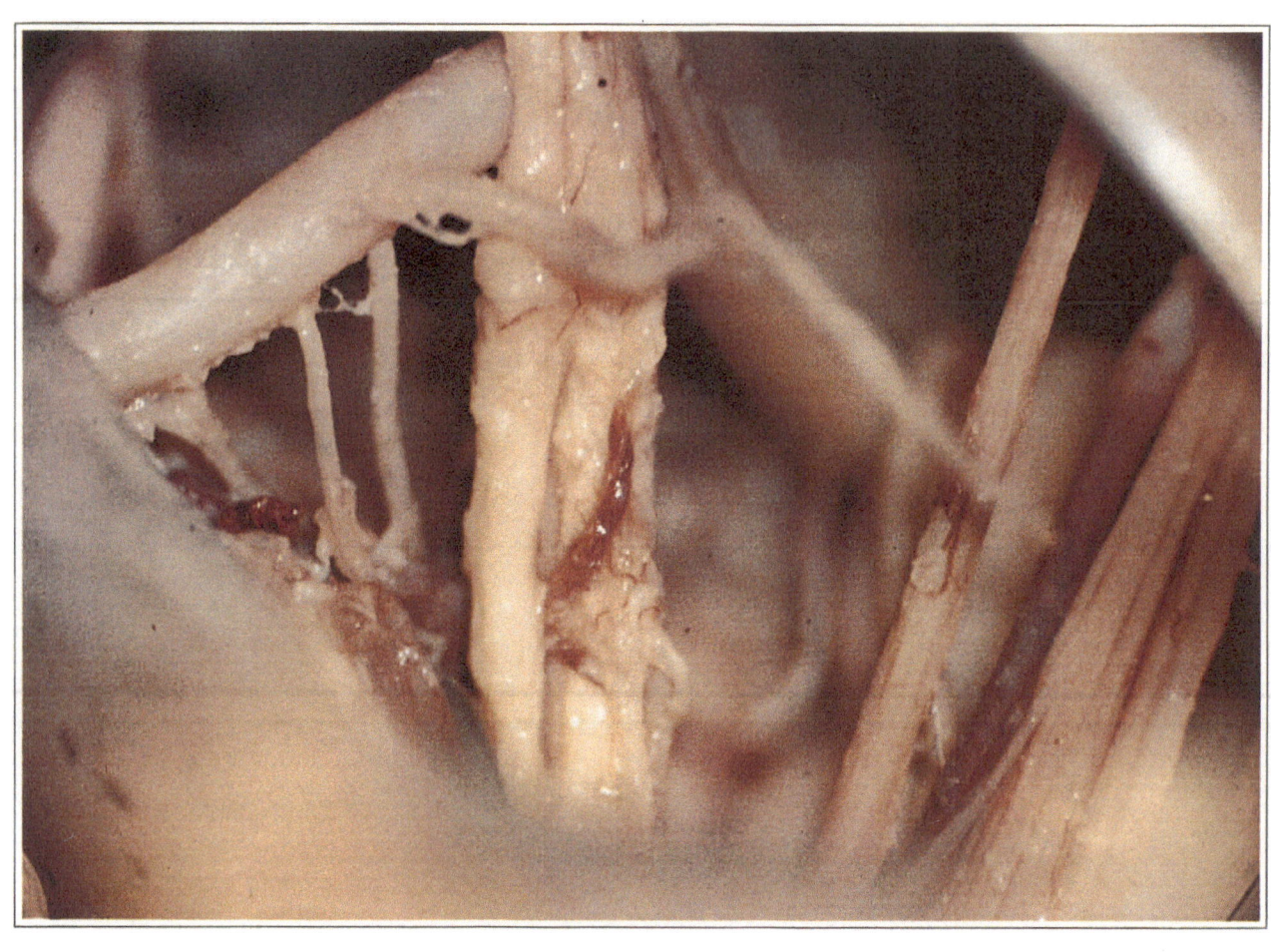

6. Close up of the VIII nerve with a loop of AICA. V is seen at the far left and IX and X at the far right.

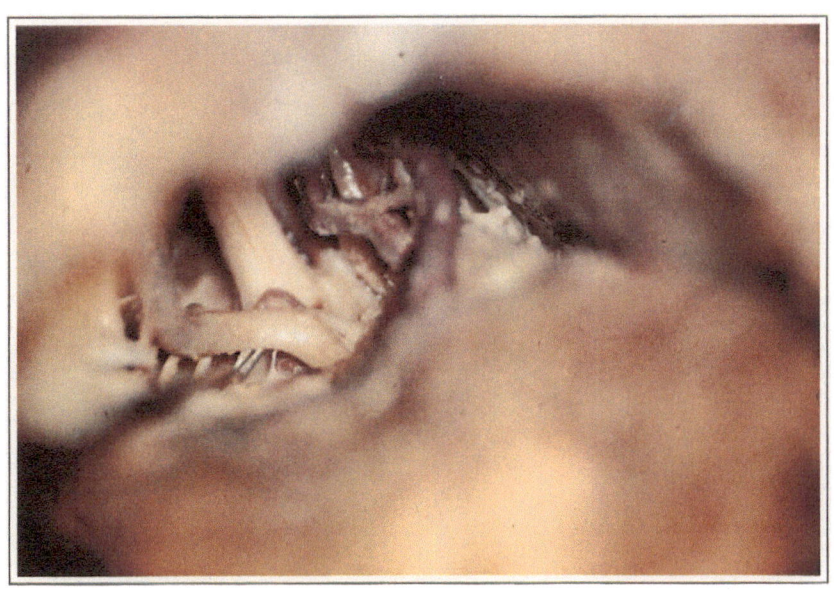

7. Close up of the root entry zone of V.

8. View of the lower cranial nerves IX, X and XI.

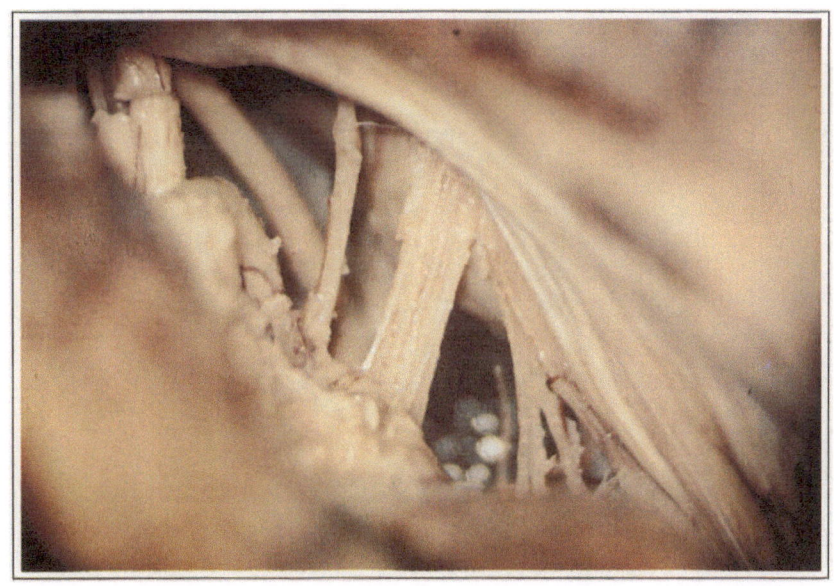

IX. TRANSCOCHLEAR APPROACH

The transcochlear approach to the skull base evolved out of the need for a transtemporal approach to lesions medial to the porus and anterior to the brainstem. The translabyrinthine route interposed the facial nerve between the surgeon and anterior temporal bone lesions. The suboccipital approach placed the cerebellum and brainstem between the operator and the tumor. Rerouting of the facial nerve allowed for total tumor removal with preservation of facial nerve function.

A. The transcochlear approach begins as a translabyrinthine procedure, performing a mastoidectomy, labyrinthectomy, and skeletonizing the facial nerve from stylomastoid foramen to IAC. The dura is left undisturbed until later.

B. The facial recess (suprapyramidal recess) is opened as in chronic ear surgery. The posterior canal wall is thinned and the chorda tympani located. The facial recess is opened by saucerizing the bone between the facial and chorda. The chorda will be sacrificed in order to extend the dissection inferiorly. As the hearing will be destroyed by drilling the cochlear turns, it is not necessary to mantain the bridge of bone at the fossa incudis. This allows for wide exposure of the facial recess. The incus is removed at this time.

C. The entire course of the facial nerve from stylomastoid to geniculate to IAC should be evident. The next part of the approach calls for meticulous dissection to mobilize the facial nerve and transpose it posteriorly.

D. With a diamond burr and copious irrigation, a trough is created on both sides of the facial nerve to access at least 180 degrees. A thin shell of bone should be left on the nerve for protection.

E. With a dental excavator, the thin shell of bone is removed from the facial nerve. The nerve is carefully elevated from the fallopian canal, starting inferiorly. The nerve is particularly tenacious near the stapedius tendon. More force must be used to free the nerve here, taking care not to avulse it.

F. When the geniculate is reached, the greater superficial petrosal nerve is identified and cut. This frees the entire length of the facial, which can now be transposed posteriorly.

G. Prior to transcochlear bone removal, the facial nerve should be protected from an errant drill. This can be accomplished by covering the nerve with cottonoids. A hardier form of protection comes from the use of the foil from a suture pack which can be cut and contoured to form a semi-conduit for the facial nerve.

H. Bone removal begins with the basal coil of the cochlea. This is drilled out until the thin septum that separates the cochlea from the internal carotid artery anteriorly is identified. The remainder of the cochlear turns are drilled out.

I. Superiorly, bone removal follows the superior petrosal sinus to Meckel's cave. Inferiorly, bone removal identifies the inferior petrosal sinus at its junction with the jugular bulb. Medially, bone removal extends into the clivus.

J. This dissection defines a triangle covered by dura. The apex is Meckel's cave. Superiorly the triangle is bounded by the superior petrosal sinus. Inferiorly, the inferior petrosal sinus forms the border.

K. The carotid artery is an important landmark. In meningiomas, there may be feeder vessels originating from the intratemporal carotid which can be controlled with a diamond burr.

L. Tumor removal is now accomplished in a fashion similar to acoustic tumor removal. The dura is opened posterior to the IAC. The opening is extended anteriorly as far as is necessary in order to identify the full extent of the tumor.

M. The relationship of the tumor to the intracranial portion of the facial nerve is assessed. The plane between the facial and tumor is developed. The tumor is gutted and its capsule removed piecemeal.

N. Hemostasis is secured with bipolar cautery prior to closure. The facial nerve is reflected anteriorly. Strips of abdominal fat are insinuated into the defect and the wound is closed in layers. It is usually not necessary to disturb the anatomy of the external auditory canal and tympanic membrane. For lesions anterior to the carotid, the external auditory canal is removed. This will be discussed in the section on infratemporal fossa surgery.

Summary: *Lesions anterior to the brainstem such as epidermoid cysts, large schwannomas or neuro-fibromas, or meningiomas can be removed by the transcochlear approach. This procedure allows the surgeon to reroute the facial nerve thereby eliminating the barrier to anterior exposure with the translabyrinthine approach. Such rerouting invariably causes some temporary facial weakness. If the nerve is anatomically intact, recovery is the rule.*

7. TRANSCOCHLEAR APPROACH

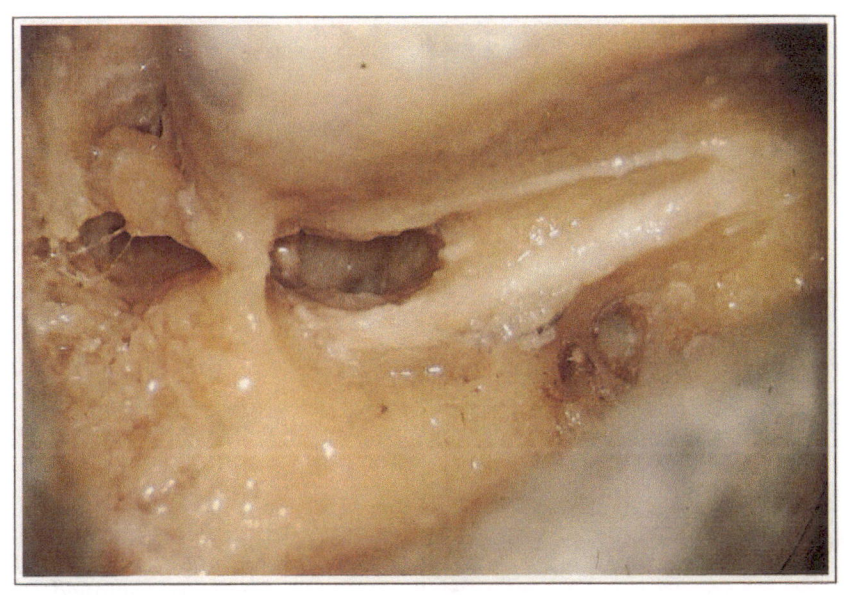

1. *A routine facial recess approach is accomplished.*

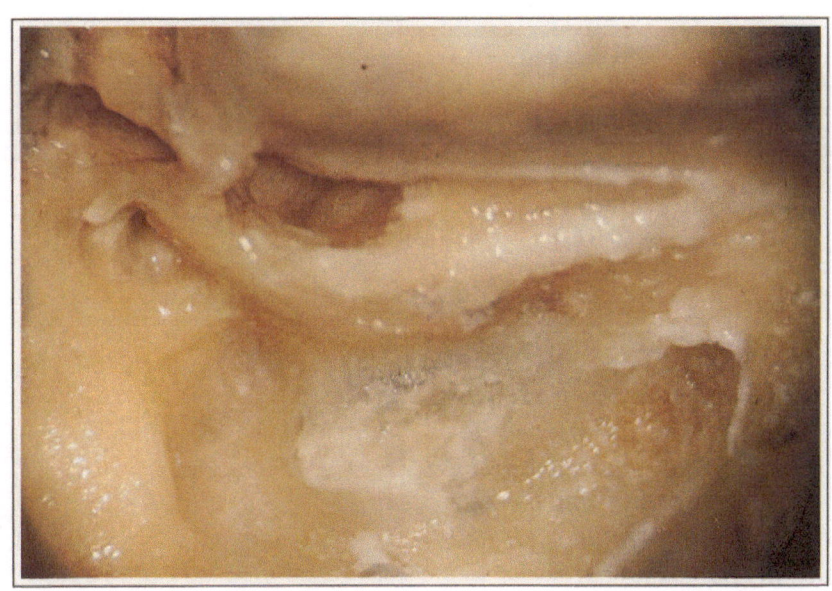

2. *The retrofacial air tract is opened exposing the endolymphatic sac.*

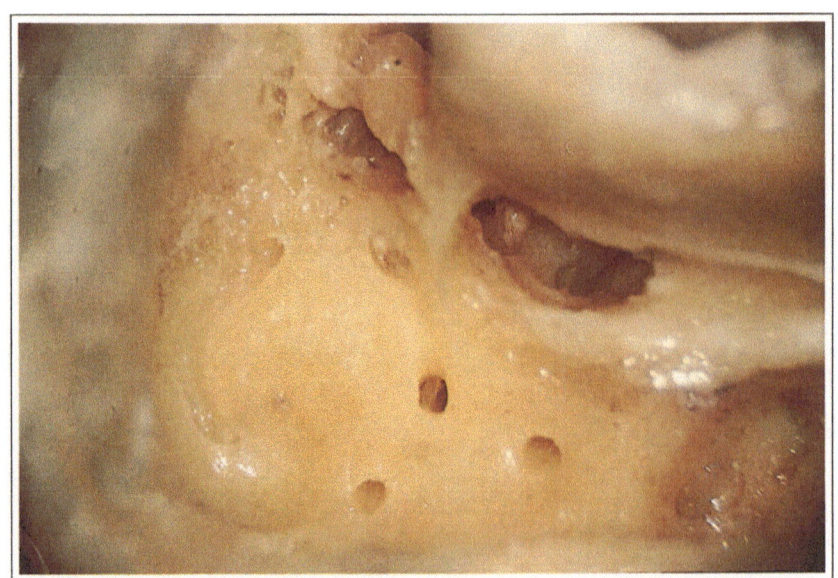

3. *A labyrinthectomy is performed.*

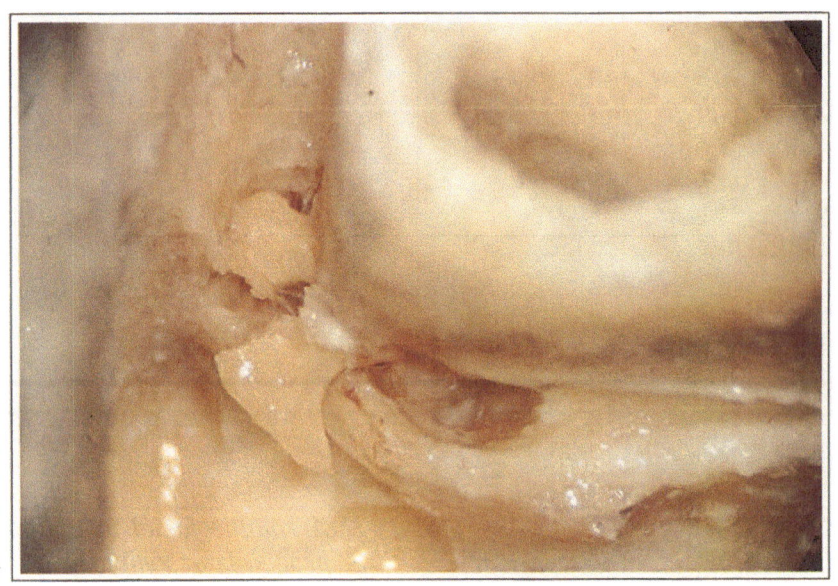

4. *The incus and malleus head are removed.*

5. *The facial nerve is skeletonized from stylomastoid foramen to geniculate. The hook is transecting the greater superficial petrosal nerve.*

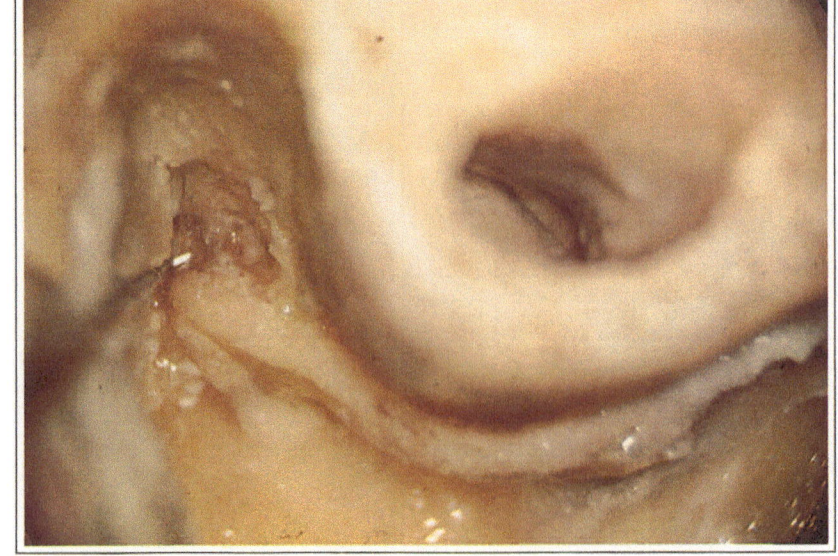

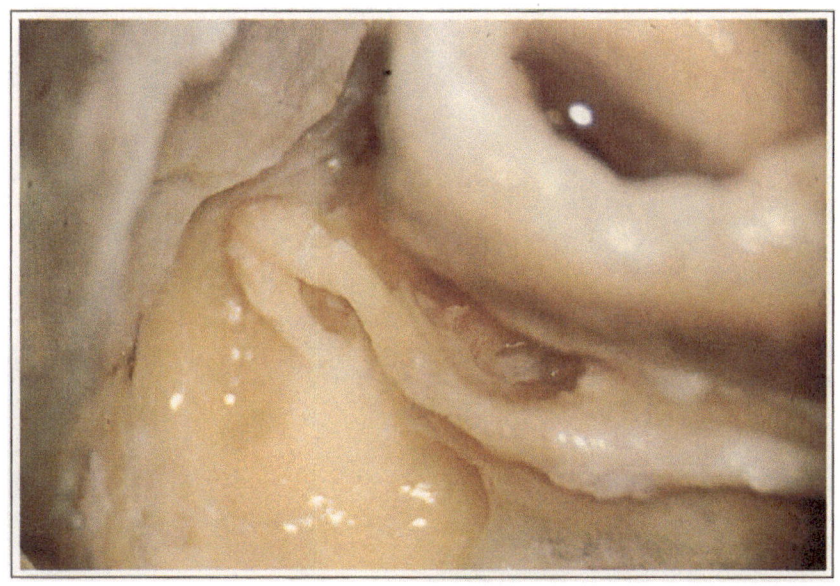

6. *The facial nerve is mobilized from the fallopian canal.*

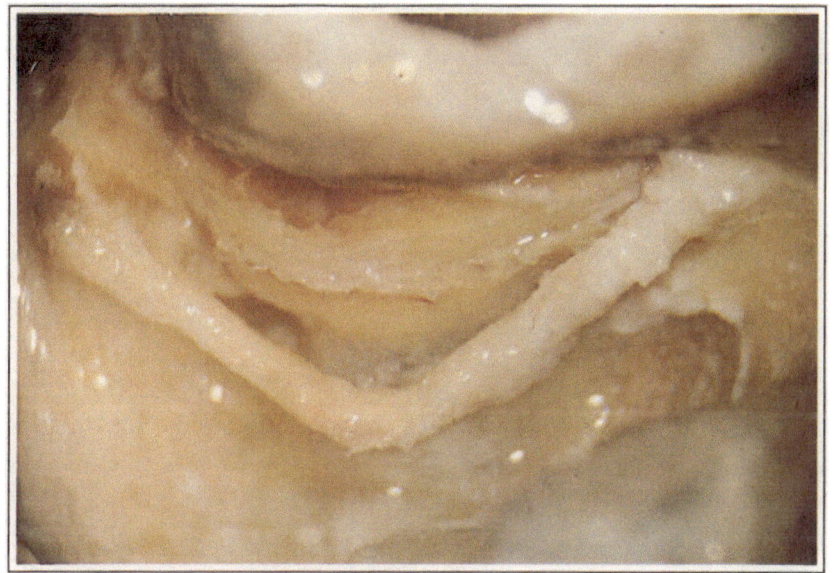

7. *The facial nerve is now re-routed posteriorly.*

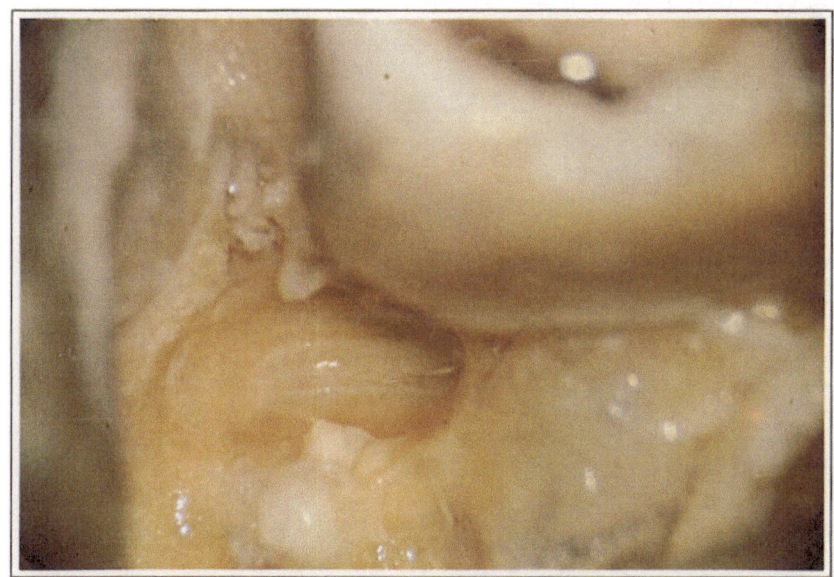

8. *With the facial rerouted, drilling proceeds deep to the nerve to expose the cochlea.*

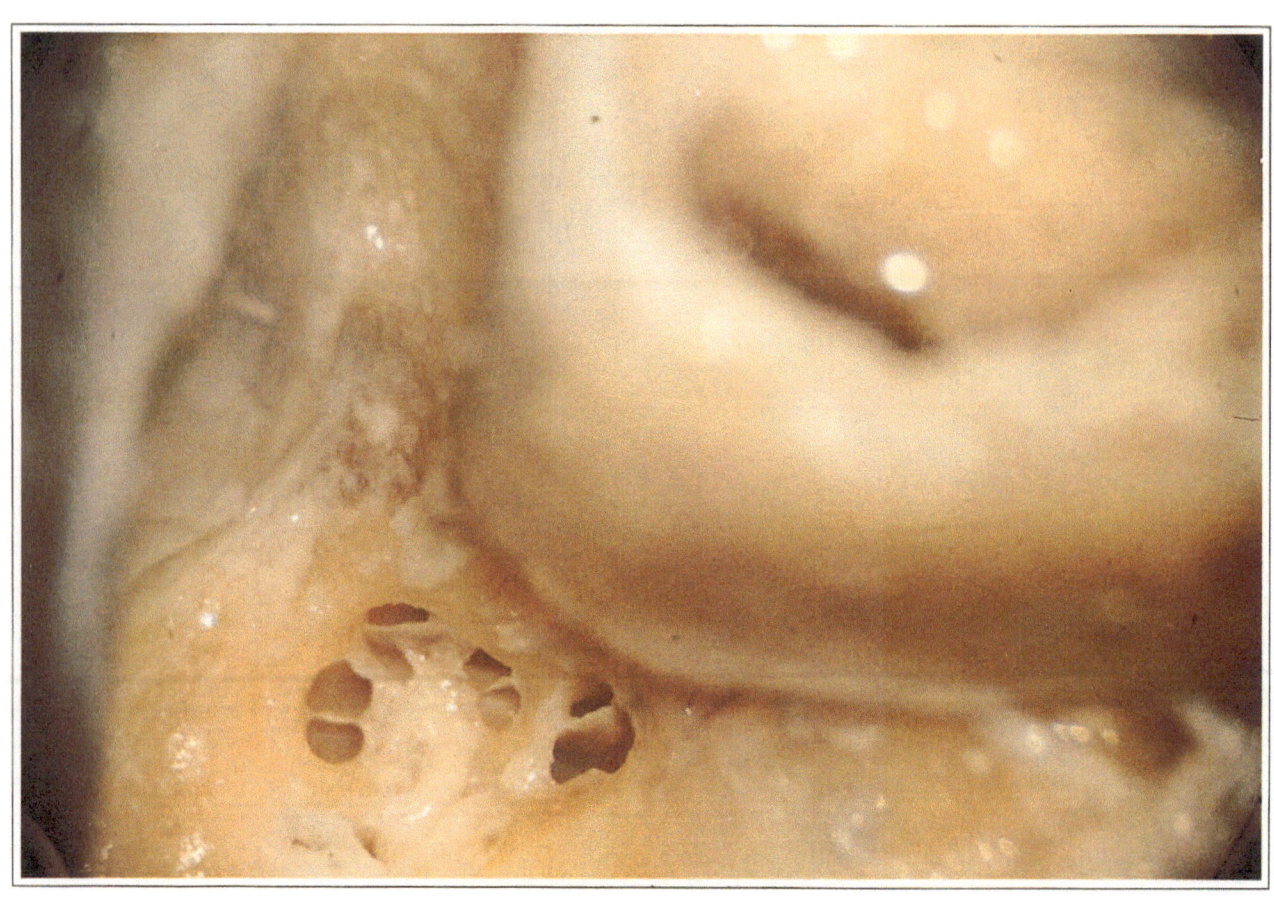

9. *The turns of the cochlea are exposed and systematically removed.*

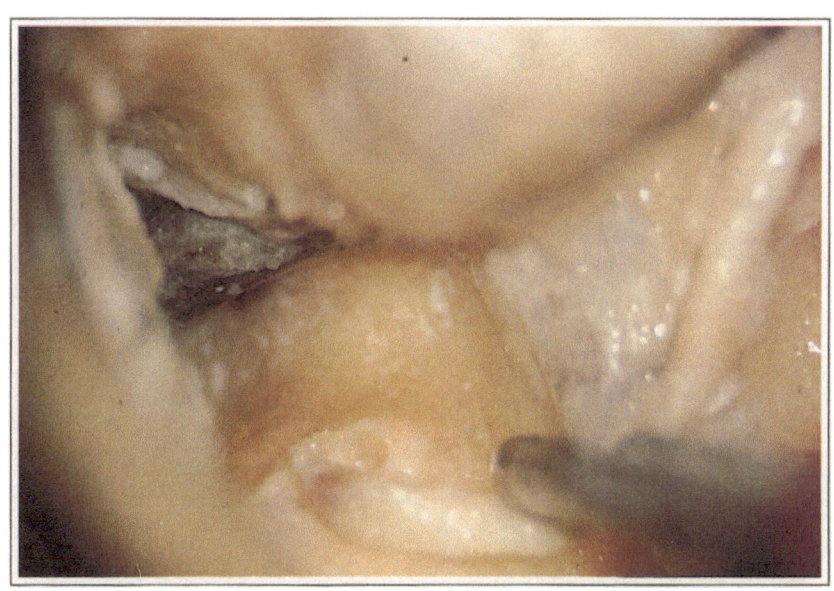

10. *Further drilling anteriorly exposes the intratemporal carotid artery. Note the jugular bulb inferiorly.*

11. *The clivus is exposed deep to the otic capsule.*

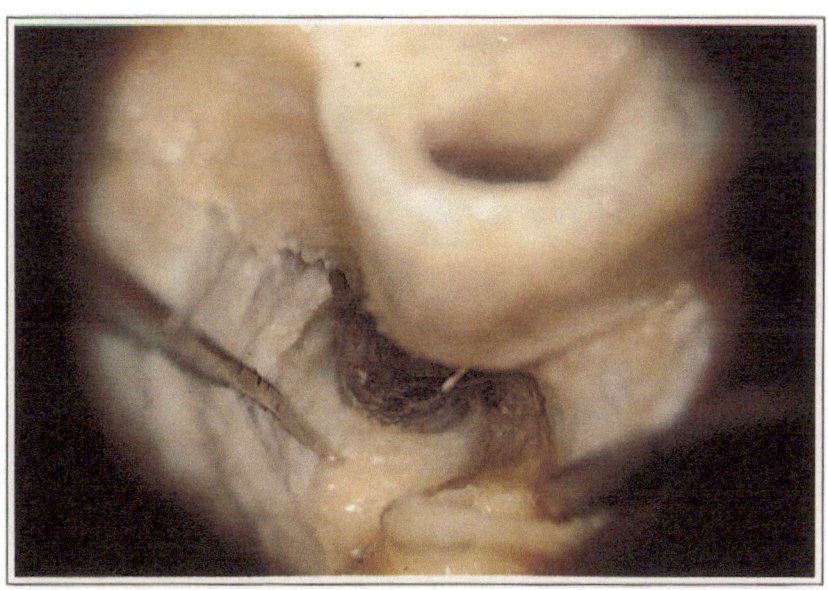

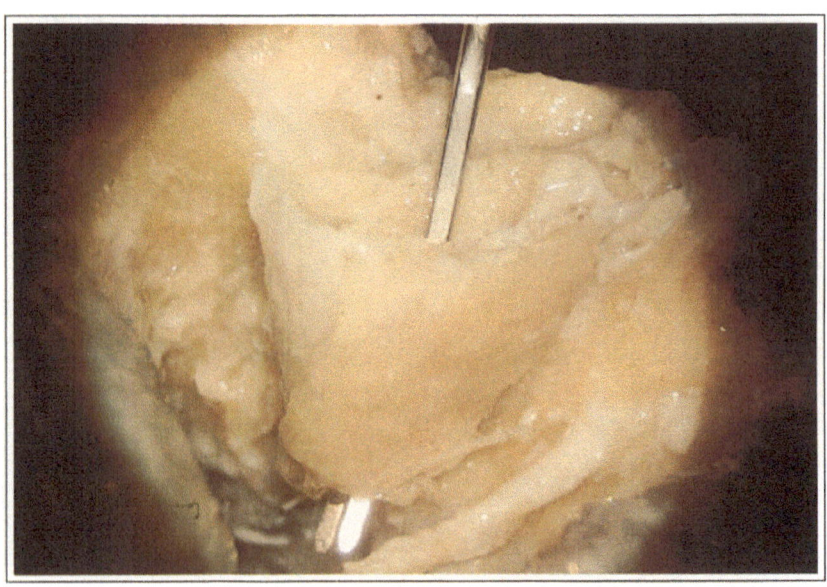

12. The external auditory canal is removed.

13. The completed dissection reveals the posteriorly displaced facial nerve, carotid artery, jugular bulb, and the jugulo-carotid spine.

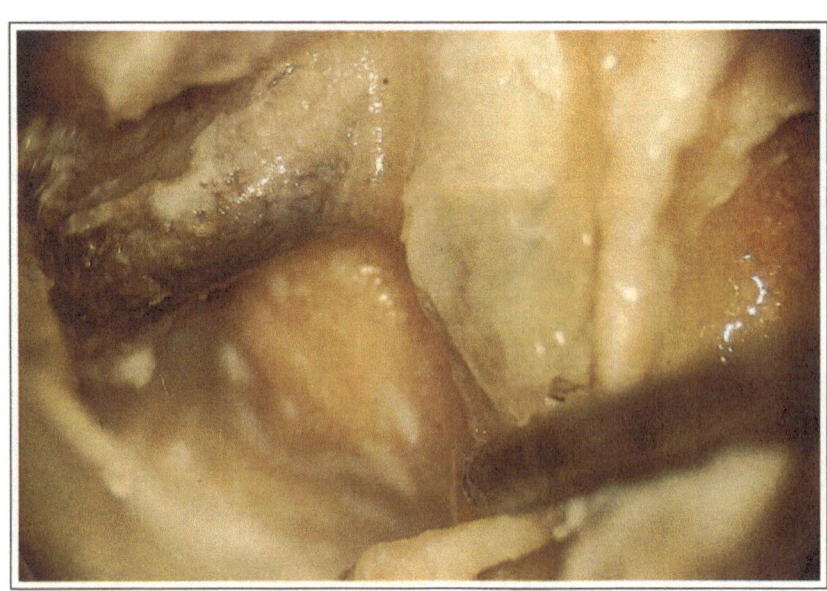

58

X. MIDDLE FOSSA SURGERY

Surgery through the middle fossa has many applications for the oto-neurological surgeon. Vestibular neurectomy can be accomplished by this route, though the authors prefer the retrolabyrinthine approach. Total facial nerve decompression and exploration can be achieved through the middle fossa. This approach also provides access to the petrous apex for the treatment of cholesterol granuloma or apicitis. And finally, small acoustic tumors can be removed via the middle fossa where preservation of hearing is desired.

A. As with other temporal bone procedures, adequate exposure begins with proper placement of the skin incision. For middle fossa surgery the surgeon sits at the head of the table and begins the incision below the zygomatic arch immediately in front of the tragus. The incision is carried cephalad with a gentle curve anteriorly, then curving posteriorly. The incision ends at about the level of the superficial temporal line, or about 8 cm from its origin.

B. The plane between the temporalis fascia and the overlying soft tissues is developed and the skin flaps are widely undermined. A large self-retaining retractor is inserted.

C. Management of the temporalis muscle depends upon the underlying condition for which the surgery is being performed. If a vestibular nerve section is to be performed, or

if the surgeon is draining a lesion of the petrous apex, situations where facial nerve injury is unlikely, then the traditional vertical muscle splitting incision may be employed. A second cut is made along the zygoma perpendicular to the first cut. The muscle is then elevated from the temporal squama.

D. For procedures where facial paralysis is already present or a likely consequence of the surgery, a different approach to the temporalis muscle should be employed. One should preserve the central 1/3 of the muscle with its neurovascular bundle. By doing this, one will be able to utilize muscle transposition techniques to reanimate the lower face in the event of an unsatisfactory facial nerve result. The authors encourage middle fossa surgeons to use this technique in all middle fossa procedures. Instead of the t-shaped incisions described above, an inferiorly based flap is created. The central 4 cm of the temporalis muscle is marked. Incisions are made down to bone on either side of this section and carried cephalad into the periosteum above the attachment of the muscle to the calvarium. The periosteum and muscle are elevated inferiorly all the way to the root of the zygoma. A traction suture can be placed in the muscle to pull it inferiorly. The remaining temporalis muscle is elevated laterally from the squama and the retractor is placed at a deeper level to expose a wide section of bone.

E. A craniotomy is now carried with a cutting burr. The bone flap is designed so that it is 1/3 posterior and 2/3 anterior to the external auditory canal. Its dimensions are roughly 3 cm x 3 cm, but can be made as large as space permits. It is most important to carry the bone removal as low as possible, removing the root of the zygoma if necessary. The inferior bone cut should be as close to the floor of the middle fossa as possible.

F. The bone flap is removed with an Adson elevator and the dura at the edges of the craniotomy elevated from the overlying bone.

G. The self-retaining House-Urban middle fossa retractor is inserted and locked onto the bone surrounding the defect. Dural dissection begins at the floor of the middle fossa and proceeds laterally to medially. If a bone ledge obscures vision of the middle fossa floor, it is removed with a rongeur.

H. Begin dural elevation anteriorly, approaching the foramen spinosum. The middle meningeal artery will be seen, and should be given wide birth. There is a menacing plexus of veins in this area which often cause troublesome bleeding.

I. The surgeon should now begin looking for the groove in the floor of the middle fossa that houses the greater superficial petrosal nerve (GSP). This is traced back to the geniculate

ganglion, which may not be protected by bone. Care should be exercised in elevating the dura here in order to avoid injury to a dehiscent geniculate.

J. Continue to elevate the dura until the arcuate eminence and petrous ridge are identified. Identify the superior petrosal sinus along the petrous ridge, taking care to avoid lacerating this structure. The superior semicircular canal is protected by the arcuate eminence. The superior canal is oriented almost directly at a right angle to the superior petrosal sinus, althougth the arcuate eminence may assume any orientation relative to the sinus. One may elect to blue-line the superior canal for positive identification.

K. With adequate exposure of the middle fossa floor, one may begin the bone removal over the geniculate with a diamond burr. The geniculate is followed into the labyrinthine segment of the facial nerve. The surgeon should keep in mind that the facial nerve will curve posteriorly and lie at a deeper level as the IAC is approached. Also, one should be aware of the basal turn of the cochlea anteriorly to the labyrinthine facial, and the ampulla of the superior canal posteriorly.

L. Follow the labyrinthine facial into the IAC. The IAC can be blue-lined now for positive identification. One must proceed with bone removal around the IAC. A diamond burr is used to create a trough anteriorly and posteriorly to the IAC until 270 degrees of bone have been removed from around the IAC. As one nears the porus medially, one is afforded more room. Near the lateral end of the IAC, keep in mind the location of the superior canal in order to avoid inadvertent fenestration.

M. For acoustic tumor removal, it is necessary to carry bone removal to the porus. This will allow access (though limited) to the posterior fossa for tumors that have slight extension beyond the porus. As in translabyrinthine surgery, leave an egg-shell layer of bone over the canal and remove it in one piece when exposure is adequate.

N. The wound is irrigated. One may now open the dura over the IAC. This is done over the posterior aspect of the canal in order to avoid the facial nerve. The dura is opened with a sharp hook and reflected to reveal the contents of the IAC. Bill's bar is palpated. If a vestibular neurectomy is to be carried out, the superior and inferior vestibular nerves are transected with a sharp hook and a diligent search for the singular nerve is undertaken.

O. For acoustic tumor removal, the superior vestibular nerve is transected. The tumor is gently rolled off of the facial, the plane being developed with a blunt hook. Extreme care must be taken to avoid interrupting the blood supply to the cochlear nerve. The tumor is rolled toward the porus until its medial extent is located. A sharp scissors transects the stump of the vestibular nerve and the tumor is removed.

P. For facial nerve surgery, the sheath of the nerve is opened into the fundus of the IAC after adequate bone removal has been accomplished. The nerve is followed into the middle ear by locating the geniculate and opening the roof of the middle ear. This should allow visualization of the cochleariform process and head of the malleus.

Q. Closure is accomplished by covering the IAC with a piece of temporalis muscle. The House-Urban retractor is removed and the temporal lobe allowed to re-expand. The bone flap is placed into the defect. The temporalis muscle flap is placed over the bone and the wound closed in layers with absorbable sutures. A Penrose drain may be placed subcutaneously and brought out of the top of the wound if there has been excessive bleeding. A standard mastoid pressure dressing is applied.

Summary: *Middle fossa surgery is usually performed with the intention of preserving hearing. It is important to have adequate exposure to the floor of the middle fossa to avoid compromise of hearing function. The anatomy can be quite variable and challenging, even to the most experienced temporal bone surgeon. The risks inherent to middle fossa surgery are slightly greater than transmastoid procedures. These include temporal lobe injury and greater chance for facial nerve compromise. The authors ask surgeons to consider the temporalis muscle sparing approach at the onset of the operation for future reanimation techniques.*

8. MIDDLE FOSSA DISSECTION *(FACIAL NERVE EXPOSURE)*

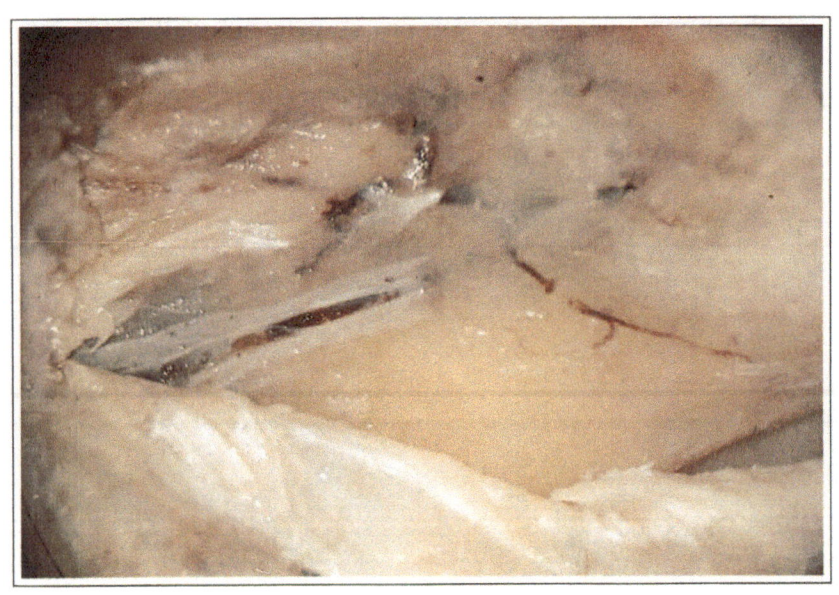

1. With the temporal lobe elevated, the greater and lesser superficial petrosal nerves are seen.

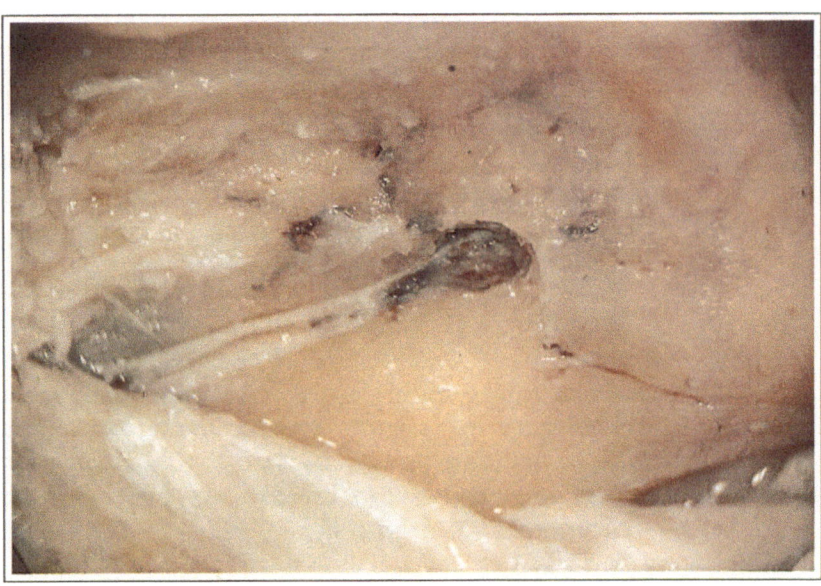

2. The geniculate ganglion area is exposed.

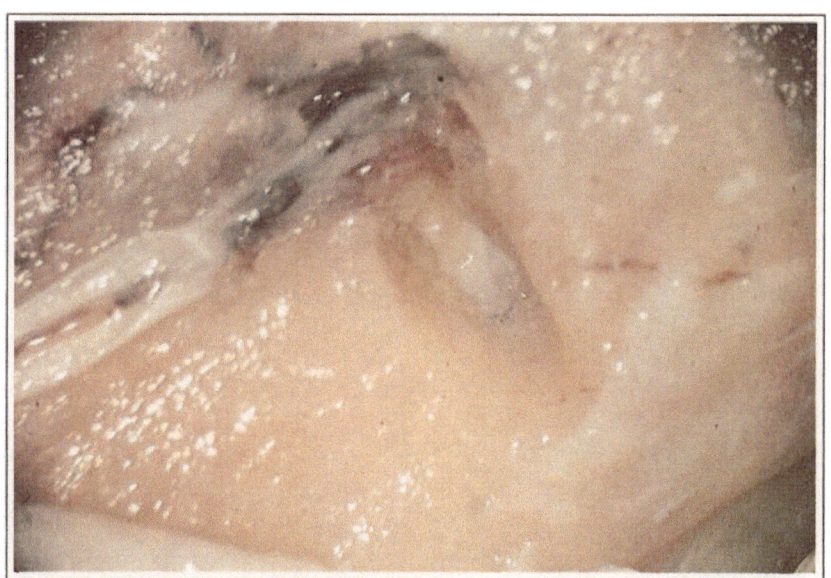

3. The geniculate ganglion is followed into the IAC.

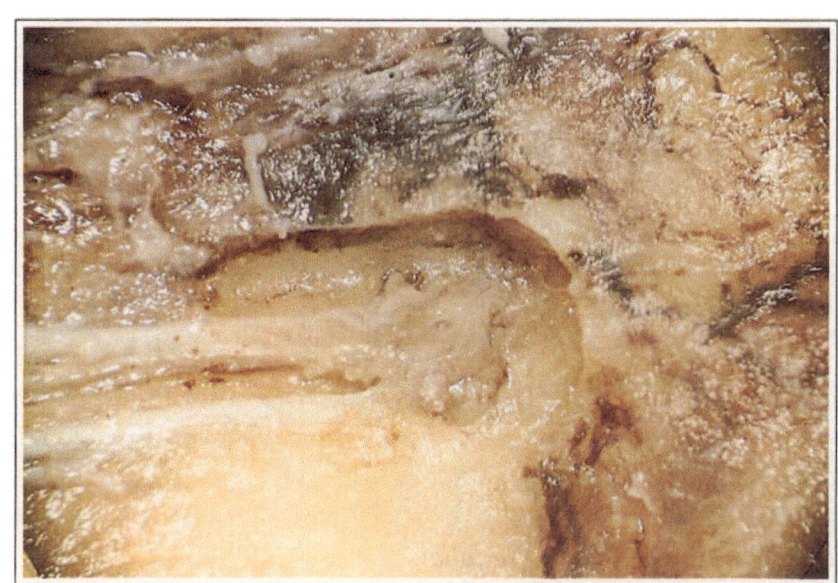

4. Close-up of the GSP and LSP and their relationship to the geniculate ganglion and IAC.

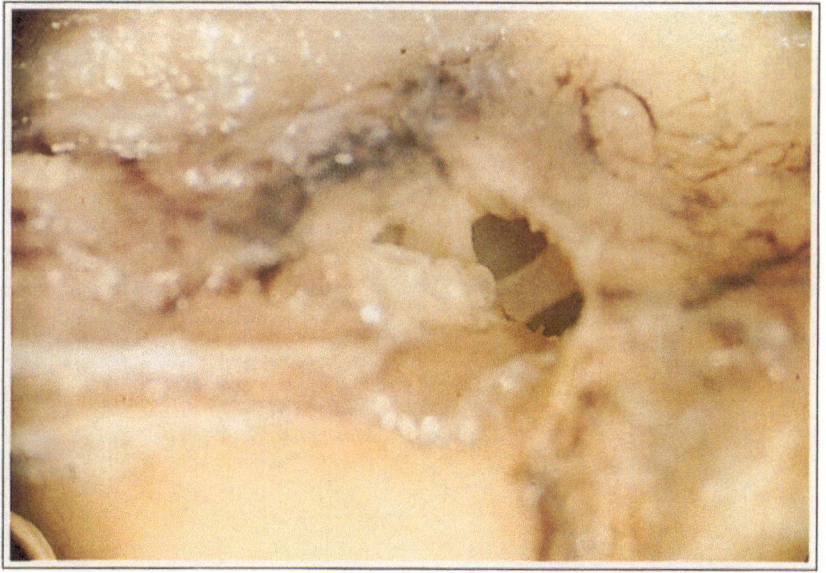

5. The roof of the epitympanum is opened revealing the tympanic portion of the facial nerve.

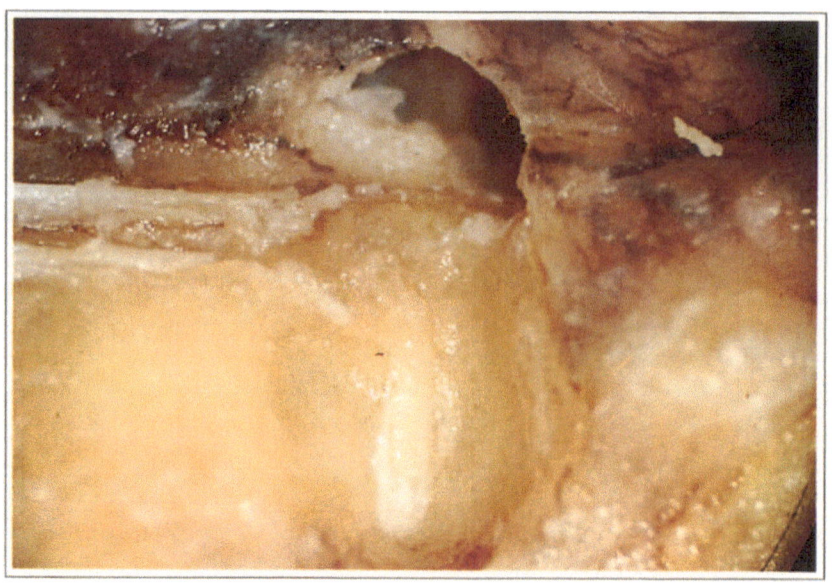

6. *Further exposure of the epitympanum reveals the head of malleus and body of incus.*

7. *The labyrinthine facial is decompressed and the nerve followed into the IAC.*

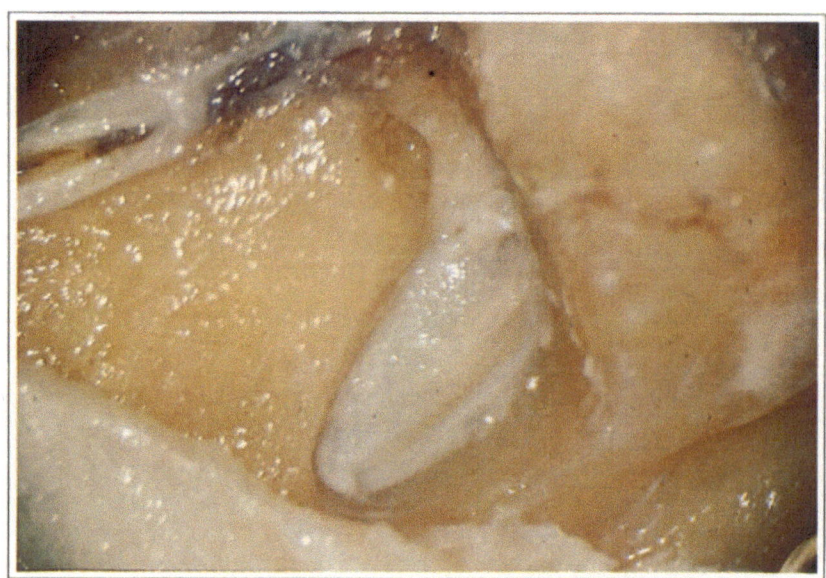

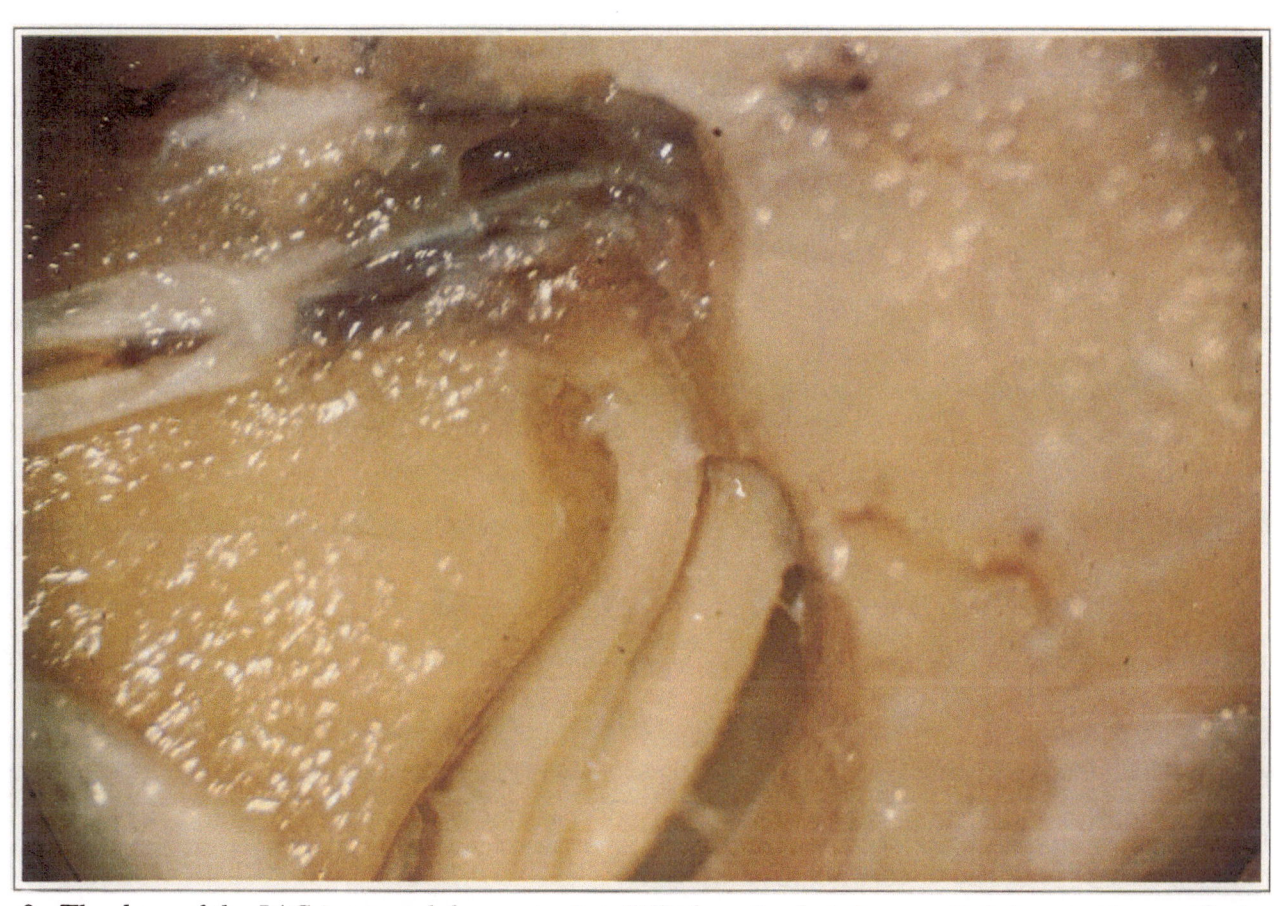

8. *The dura of the IAC is opened demonstrating Bill's bar, the facial nerve, and the superior vestibular nerve.*

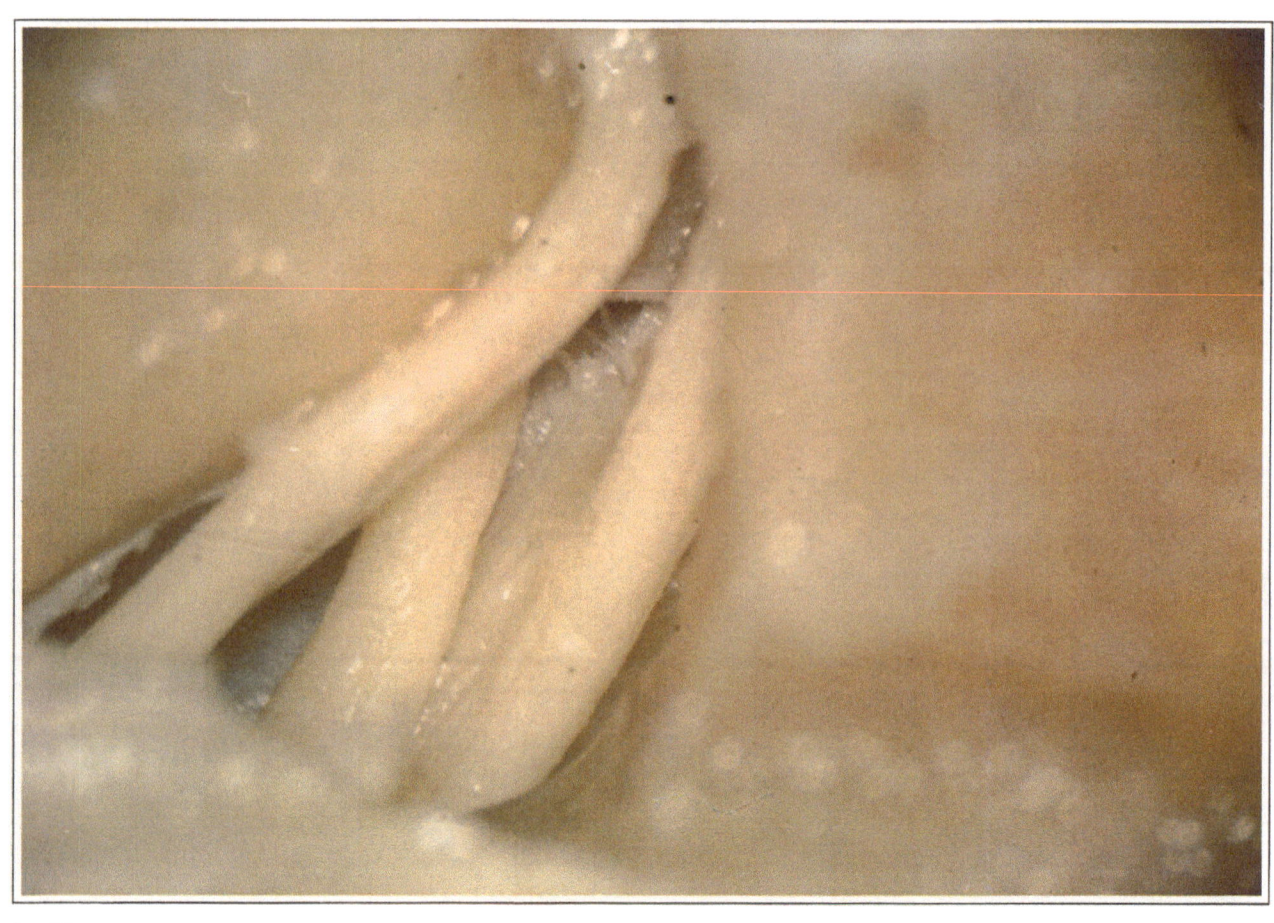

9. *The vestibulofacial fibers have been cut and all of the nerves of the IAC are well seen.*

9. MIDDLE FOSSA DISSECTION *(VESTIBULAR NERVE SECTION)*

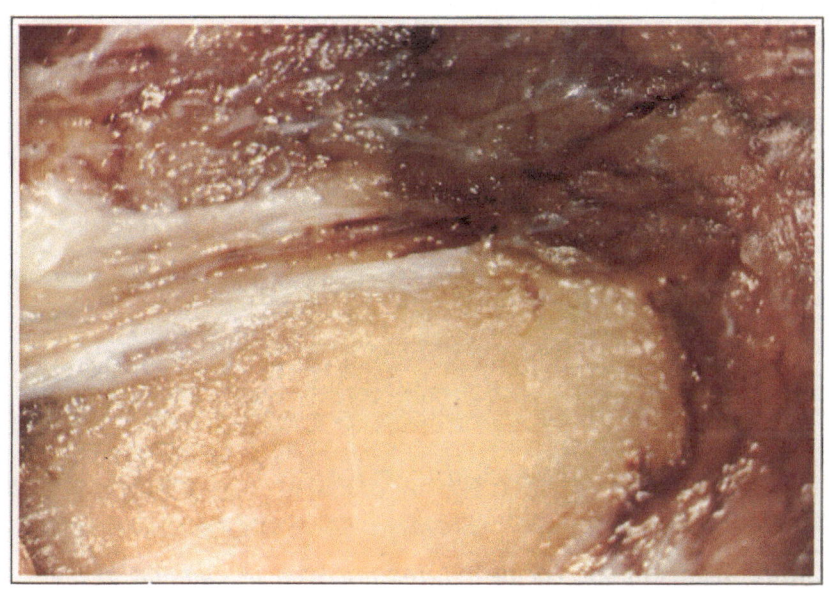

1. *The temporal lobe is elevated from the floor of the middle fossa and both greater and lesser superficial petrosal nerves are identified.*

2. *Both greater and lesser superficial petrosal nerves are seen. The basal turn of the cochlea and the superior semicircular canal are opened for reference. The IAC and geniculate ganglion are also seen.*

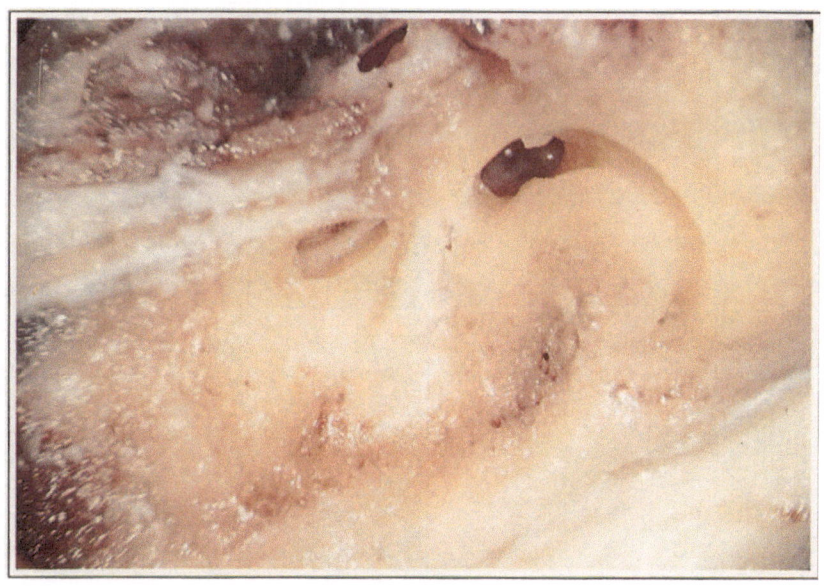

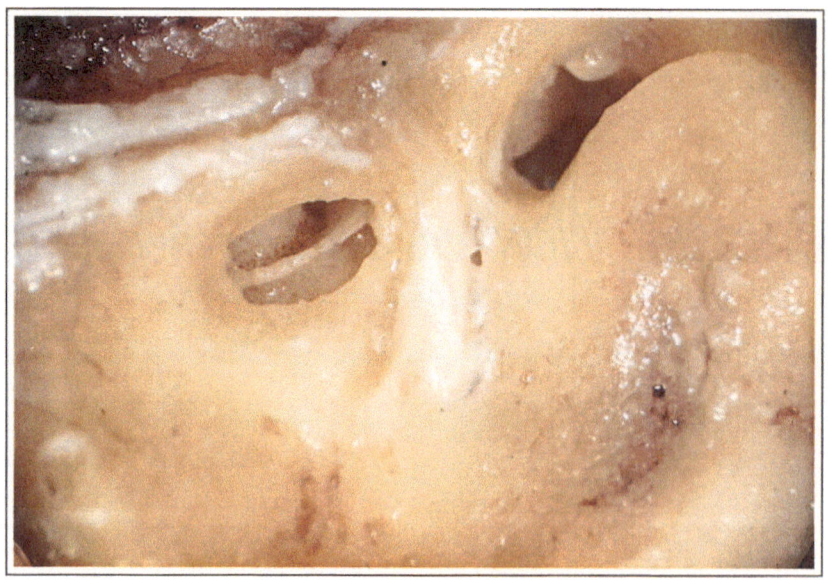

3. *The cochlear turns are seen in reference to the labyrinthine portion of the facial nerve.*

4. *More details of the cochlear turns are seen in addition to the superior vestibular nerve and Bill's bar.*

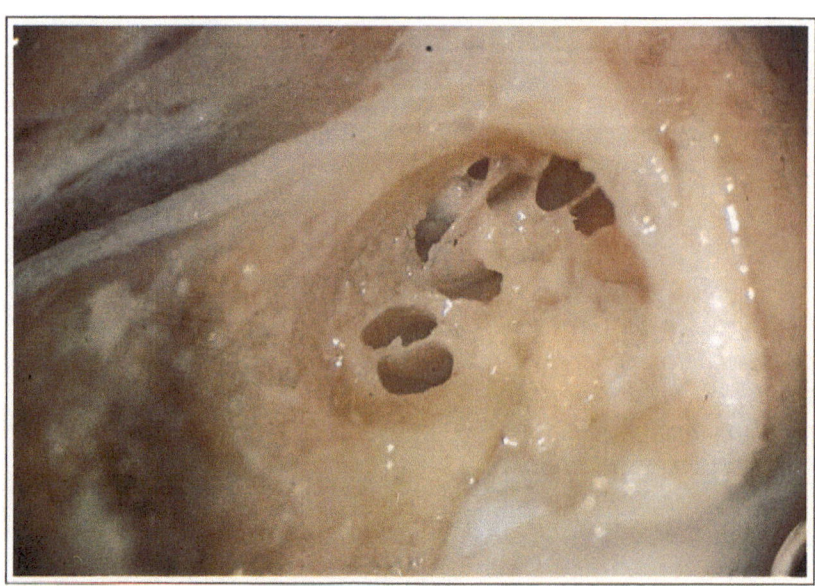

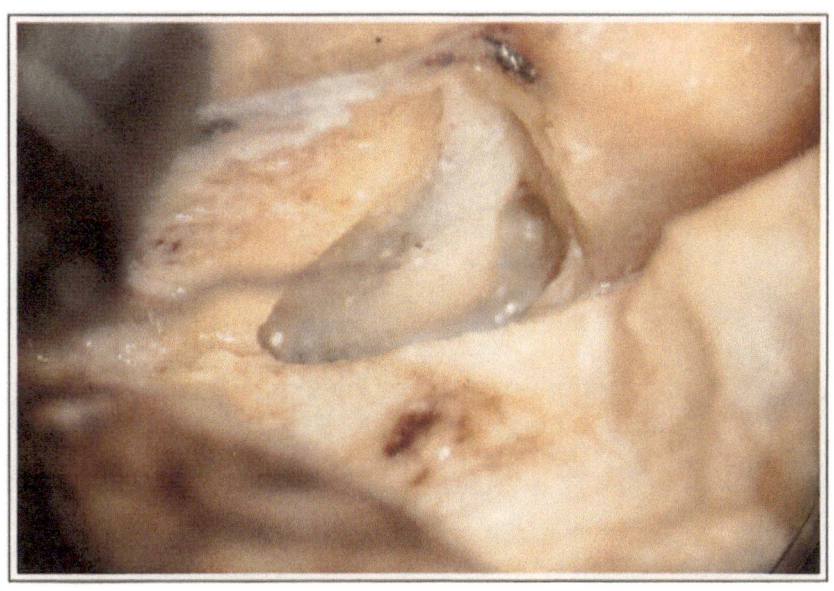

5. More bone is removed over the IAC.

6. The IAC is widely skeletonized and the dura opened. The contents of the IAC are well visualized.

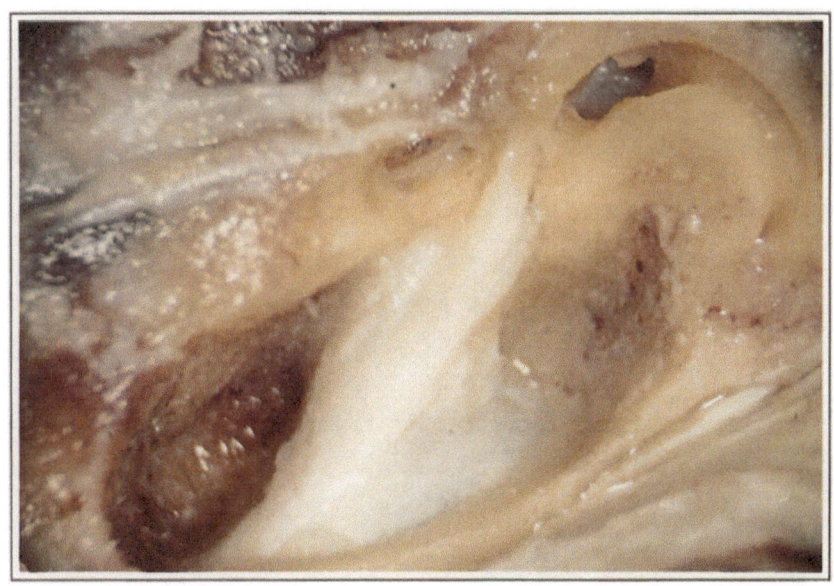

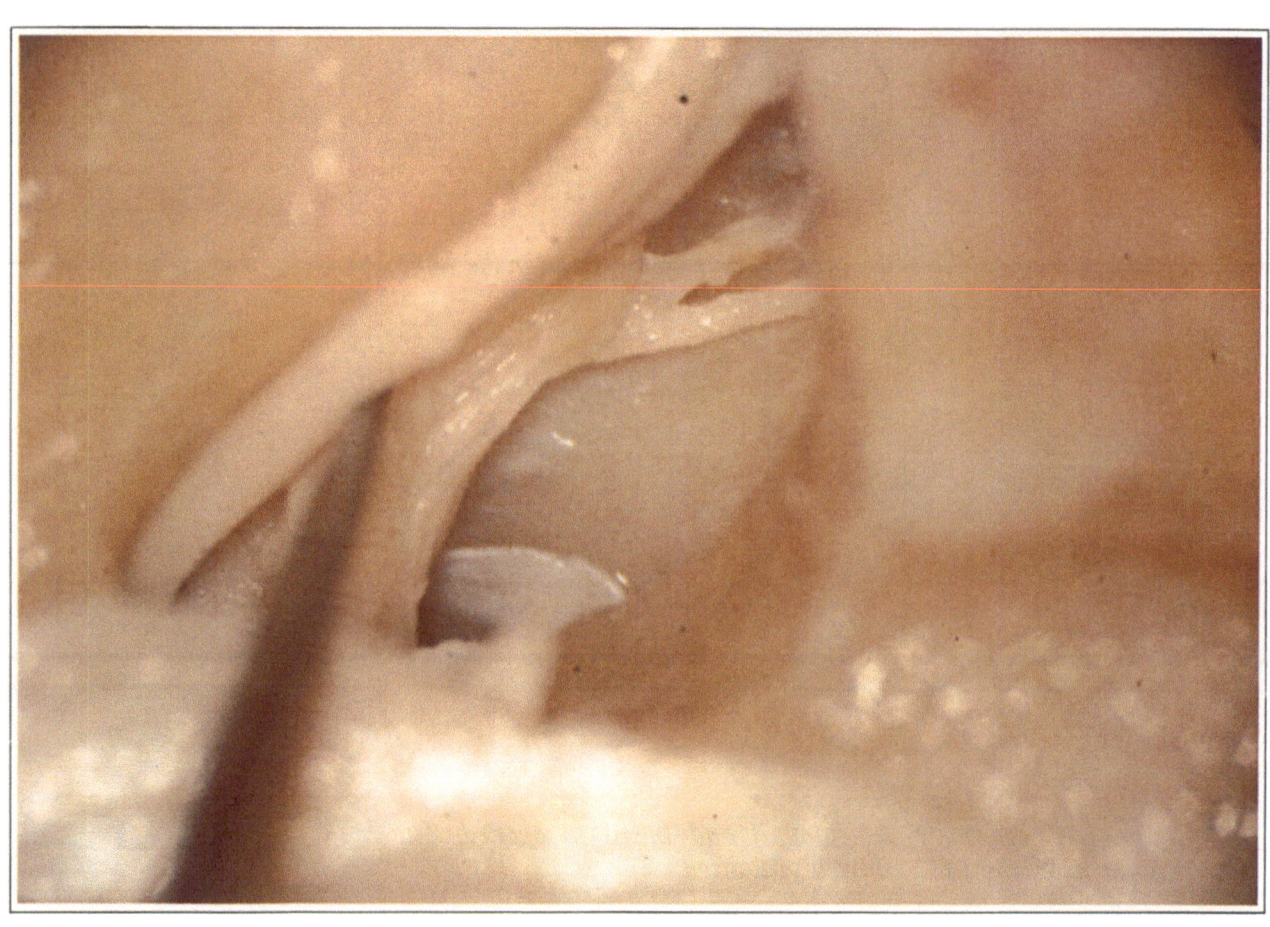

7. *Superiorly, the facial nerve is seen. With the superior vestibular cut and reflected, the inferior vestibular nerve and singular nerve are seen.*

XI. INFRATEMPORAL FOSSA APPROACH

The infratemporal fossa approach was designed to provide access to the skull base for resection of large glomus tumors and other lesions of the jugular foramen area. The facial nerve is rerouted anteriorly to provide direct access to the jugular foramen and adjacent skull base. This approach can allow the surgeon to control the intratemporal portion of the carotid artery and follow it to the parasellar area. Transcochlear extention of this approach provides access to the clivus and areas medial to the carotid.

A. Preparation of the patient for infratemporal fossa surgery requires careful planning and a team approach combining the talents of oto-neurologist, neurosurgeon, head and neck surgeon, anesthesiologist, and internist. The entire hemicranium and ipsilateral neck must be prepared and draped. A urinary catheter is inserted for monitoring urinary output. Arterial blood pressure is monitored via an arterial line. An indwelling lumbar subarachnoid catheter is placed to provide CSF drainage postoperatively to reduce the chance for CSF leakage.

B. The skin incision for infratemporal fossa surgery is placed 4 cm behind the postauricular sulcus. It begins in the area of the temporalis squama above the auricle and curves behind the ear and mastoid. It continues into the neck coursing along the posterior border of the sternocleidomastoid muscle (SCM) and curves forward following a natural skin crease.

C. The incision is carried down to the temporalis muscle. A cut is made down to the bone along the linea temporalis, taking care not to cut into the temporalis. Just behind the external auditory canal, a rectangular musculo-periosteal flap is created which will be sutured over the transected external auditory canal (EAC) to permanently close the meatus.

D. The incision can now be carried down to bone along the mastoid toward the tip. Soft tissues, including the rectangular musculo-periosteal flap are elevated from the cortex until the spine of Henle is identified. The EAC is transected at this point.

E. Prior to continuing the dissection into the neck, the surgeon closes the external auditory meatus at this time. The cartilage is dissected in a retrograde fashion, preserving skin and soft tissues. At the superior and inferior ends of the meatus a 2.0 silk suture is passed. The suture is then brought out through the meatus so as to evert it. The everted meatus is closed with interrupted 2.0 silk sutures. The musculo-periosteal flap is closed over the internal part of the meatus with 2.0 chromic sutures.

F. The incision in the neck is now developed by creating superior and inferior flaps as in a neck dissection. The trapezius should be seen posteriorly and the mandible anteriorly/superiorly. The elevation of the skin flap should be continued to the face in order to identify the lateral lobe of the parotid gland.

G. For wide access to neurovascular structures in the neck, the authors prefer to carry out a modified upper neck dissection at this time. The internal jugular vein (IJV) is isolated and followed to the skull base. A vessel loop is placed around the IJV for control. Likewise, the carotid artery and cranial nerves IX, X, and XI are isolated and traced to the skull base. To facilitate this exposure, the SCM is detached from the mastoid tip and reflected inferiorly. The posterior belly of the digastric is detached and reflected anteriorly. As much soft tissue as possible is removed from the mastoid at this time. The transverse process of C I should be easily identifiable.

H. The surgeon identifies the tympanomastoid fissure and locates the extratemporal facial nerve as in a parotidectomy. The facial is traced to its bifurcation.

I. The large flap of soft tissue elevated from the temporalis is sutured forward out of the way. The middle portion of the temporalis muscle is isolated as described earlier and mantained on its pedicle at the zygomatic arch. This temporalis muscle flap can be reflected forward and sutured to the skin flap to protect it. Again, this temporalis sparing maneuver will allow the surgeon flexibility in facial reanimation techniques if needed later.

J. Self-retaining retractors are inserted and the bone work begins. A complete mastoidectomy is performed. The sigmoid is decompressed, as are the middle and posterior fossa plates. The retrofacial air tract is opened widely. The facial nerve is located and traced to the stylomastoid foramen. The facial recess is opened. The bone over the fossa incudis can be drilled away and the incus removed. The facial recess dissection is extended inferior to the annulus sacrificing the chorda tympani nerve. The surgeon should now have good hypotympanic exposure.

K. With the facial nerve now well-outlined in the temporal bone and the parotid gland, the boney EAC can be removed with a cutting burr. No attempt is made to dissect away the skin, it is simply drilled away. The tympano-mastoid joint (TMJ) is blue-lined anteriorly.

L. With the facial still covered with bone, the mastoid tip is removed with a rongeur. The tympanic ring is drilled away anteriorly down to the level of the facial nerve. Further removal of soft tissue at the skull base allows better visualization of the IJV, carotid, and nerves VII, IX, X, and XI.

M. The sigmoid is followed with a diamond until the jugular bulb is seen. This is now skeletonized and decompressed. Part of the bulb will be obscured by the facial.

N. The facial nerve is now decompressed to the level of the geniculate by creating troughs on either side of the nerve and removing the last remnants of bone with a dental excavator. Mobilize the nerve preserving the sheath. Mobilization is most difficult at stylomastoid foramen and near the stapedius. Once totally free, the nerve is transposed anteriorly.

O. The final obstacle of the jugular foramen and skull base is now out of harm's way. With a diamond burr, the remainder of the bone over the bulb is removed. The crest (if not destroyed by tumor) between the jugular and carotid is now seen. For resection of glomus tumors, the surgeon will ligate the IJV in the neck. The sigmoid will be packed extraluminally with surgicel near the sino-dural angle. The jugular bulb and IJV can be resected en bloc. Brisk bleeding will ensue from the orifice of the inferior petrosal sinus. This is plugged with muscle and packed with surgicel. This inevitably leads to compromise of cranial nerves IX and X and to a lesser extent, XI.

P. For intracranial extention, the posterior fossa dura can be opened. Access to the clivus will be afforded by transcochlear extension of the dissection, taking care to follow the course of the carotid artery. Translabyrinthine dissection may be required to chase intracranial tumor.

Q. Closure is accomplished obliterating the defect with abdominal fat. The central portion of the temporalis is returned to its normal portion for potential future use. The rest of the temporalis can be used to help obliterate the defect. A drain connected to suction is placed in the neck. A nasogastric tube is placed for feeding. For large tumors with compromise of the nerves of the jugular foramen, and especially in elderly patients, a decision must be made now regarding tracheotomy. If there is any doubt as to the patient's ability to handle secretions, the surgeon must perform a tracheotomy prior to extubation.

Summary: *The infratemporal fossa dissection provides access to the skull base by anterior transposition of the facial nerve. Adequate exposure in the neck is of paramount importance for tumor control. Extension of tumor into the posterior fossa and clivus can be managed by modifying this approach. The extent of this surgery and its attendant morbidity and mortality mandates thorough preoperative counseling and a well-coordinated surgical effort by an experienced team.*

10. INFRATEMPORAL FOSSA DISSECTION

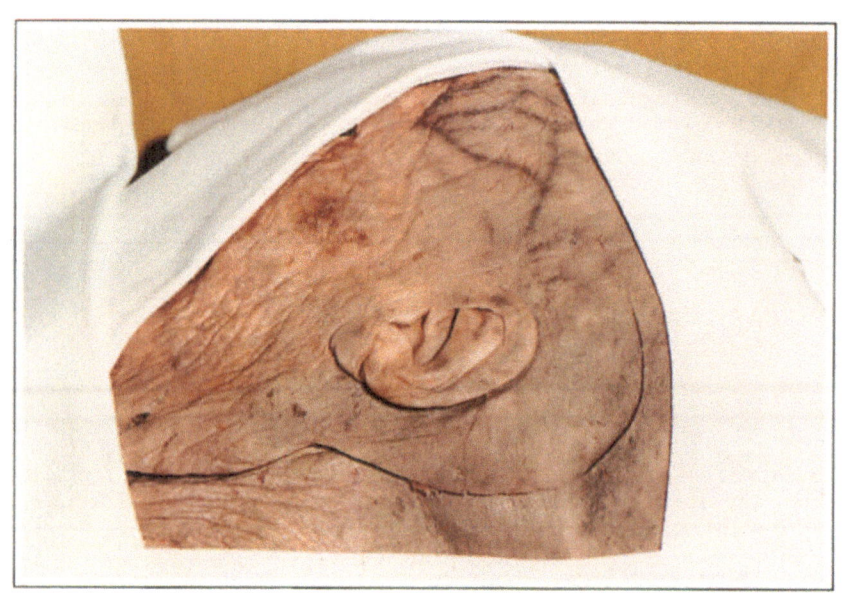

1. *The field is prepared, draped, and the skin incision outlined.*

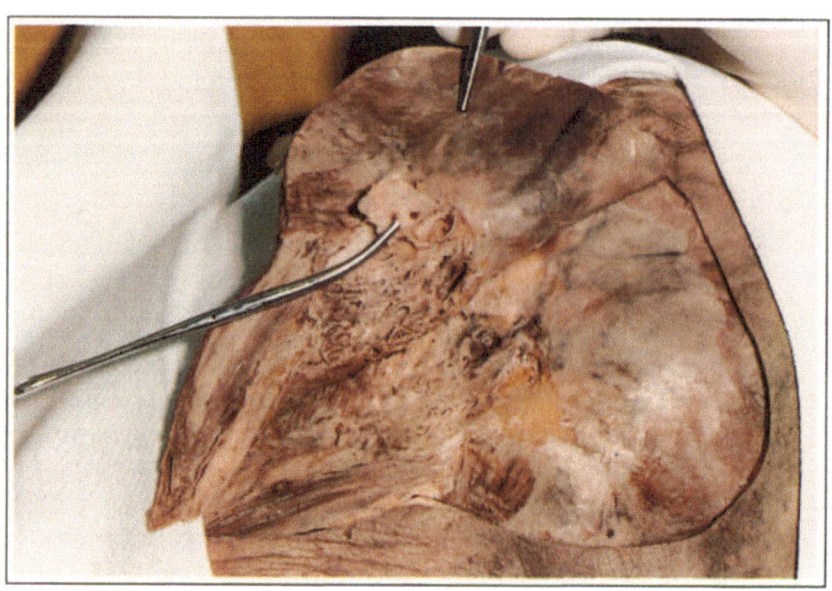

2. *The skin flap is elevated, creating a periosteal flap to close the external auditory canal.*

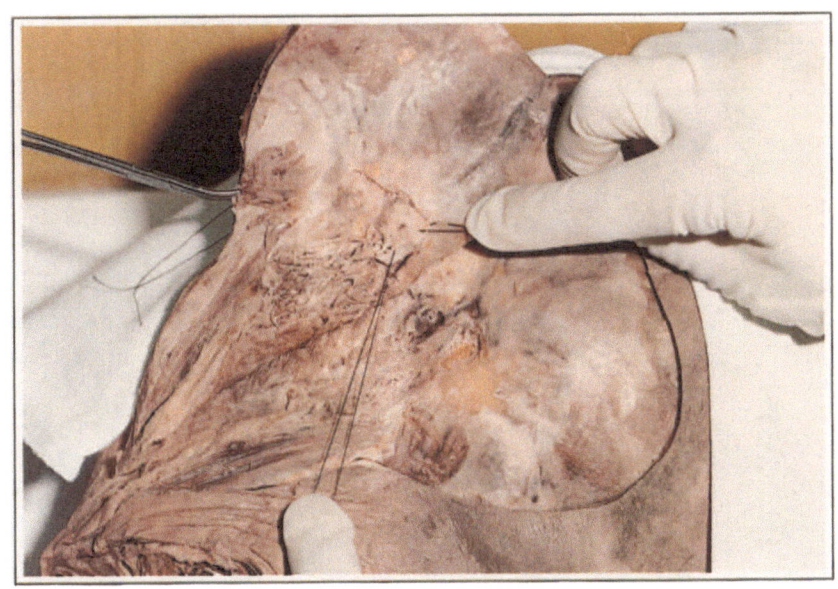

3. The EAC is closed internally with the periosteal flap.

4. The central portion of the temporalis muscle is preserved so that it can be used for a reanimation technique.

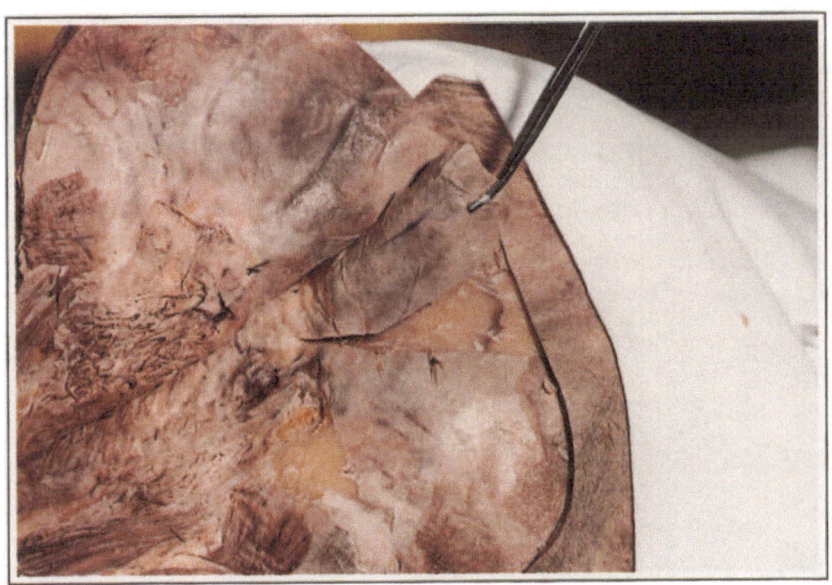

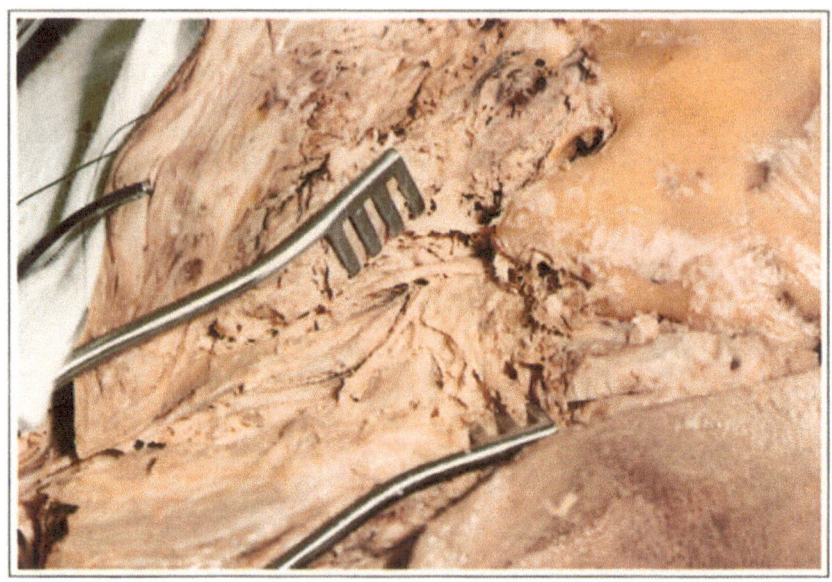

5. *The upper neck dissection is complete, identifying the jugular vein, carotid artery, and nerves X and XI.*

6. *The pointer identifies XI nerve.*

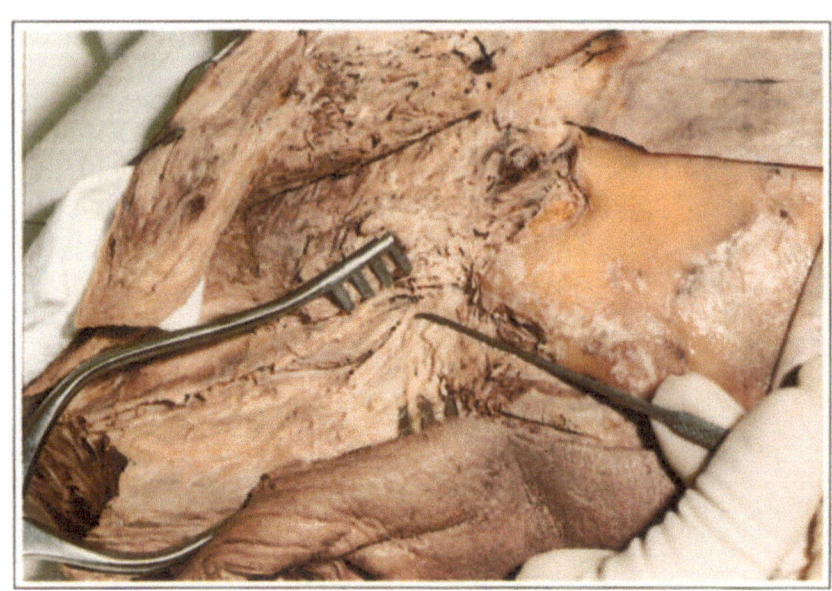

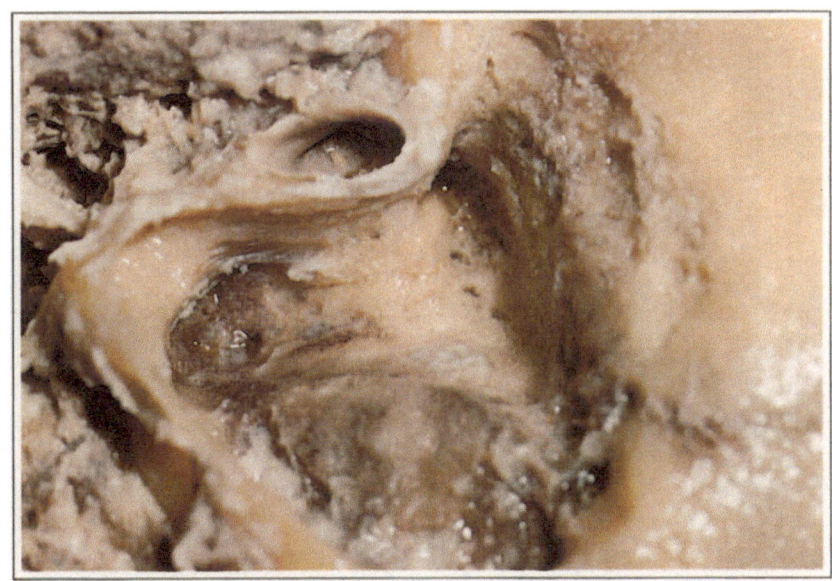

7. *A complete mastoidectomy is performed.*

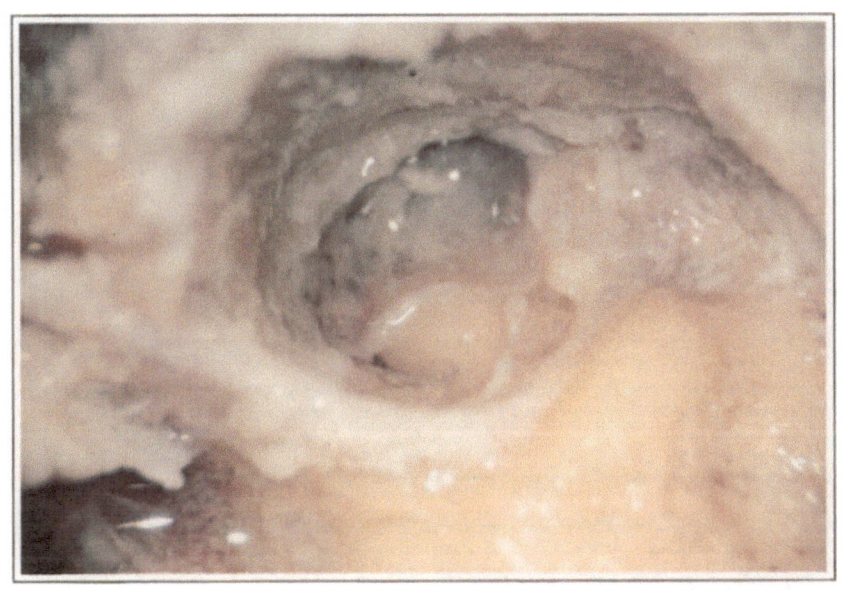

8. *The external auditory canal is removed and the facial nerve identified.*

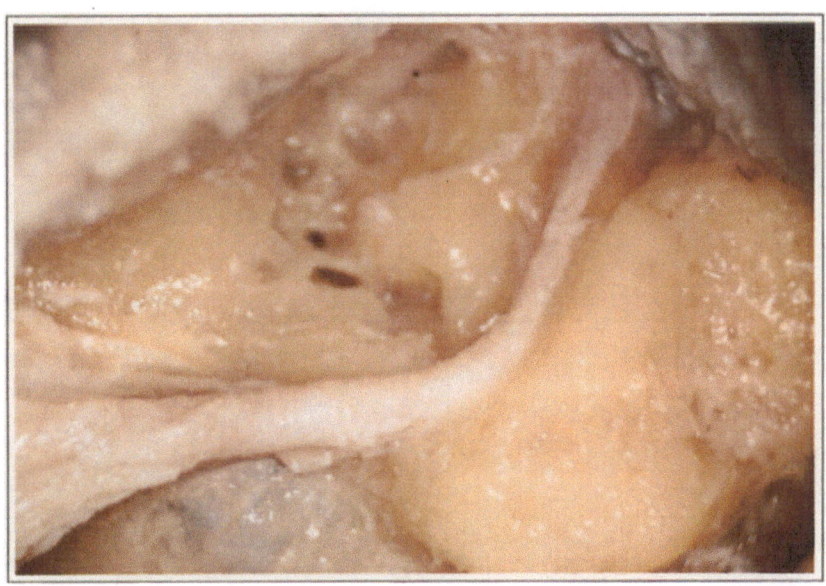

9. *The facial nerve is skeletonized from geniculate to stylomastoid foramen.*

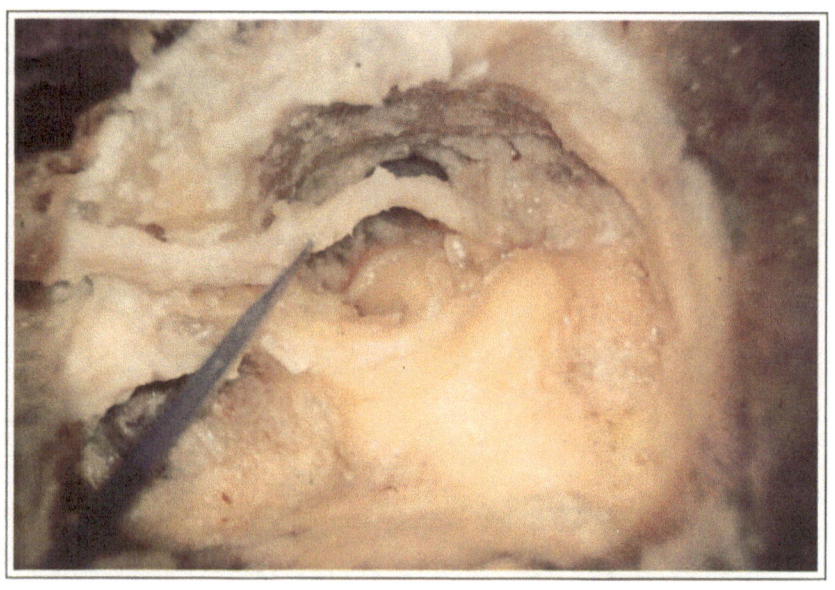

10. *The facial nerve is mobilized and transposed anteriorly.*

11. *The facial nerve is traced to the bifurcation and pes anserinus.*

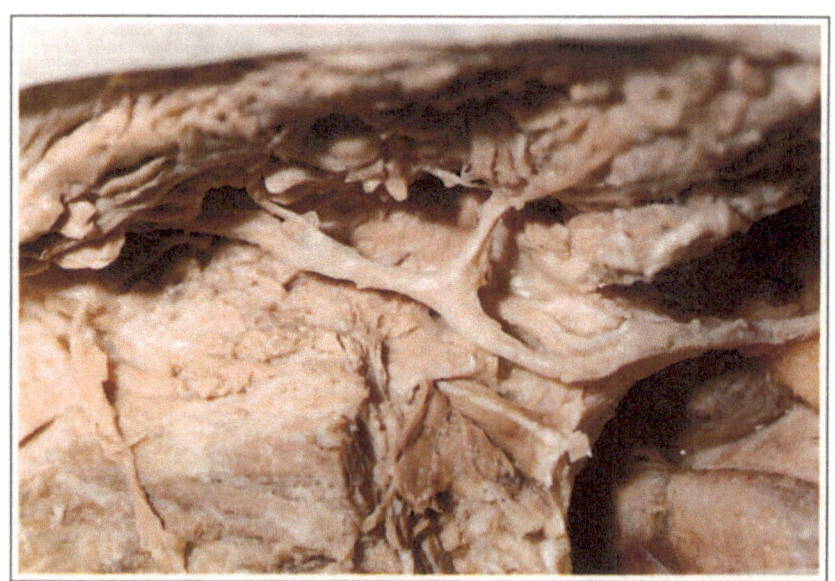

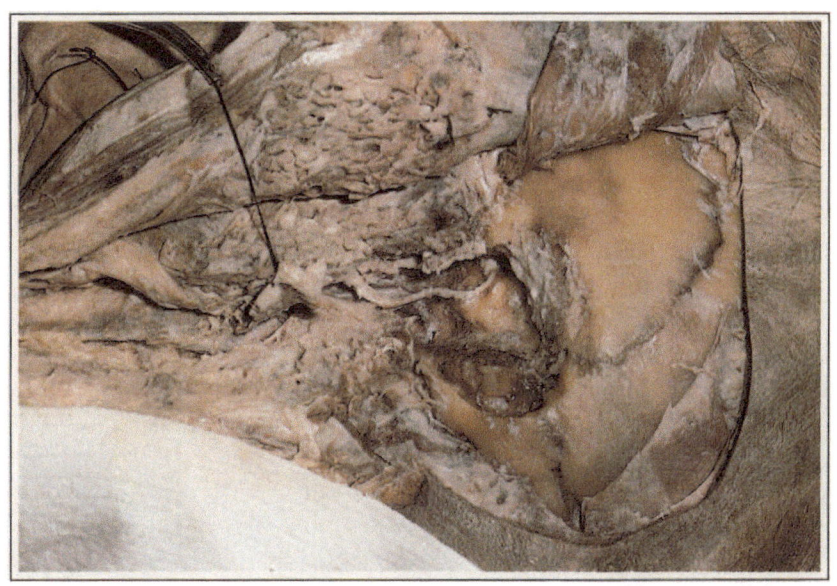

12. The limits of dissection can be seen in this picture.

13. Further exposure of the posterior fossa dura and opening the dura to remove intracranial extension of the tumor.

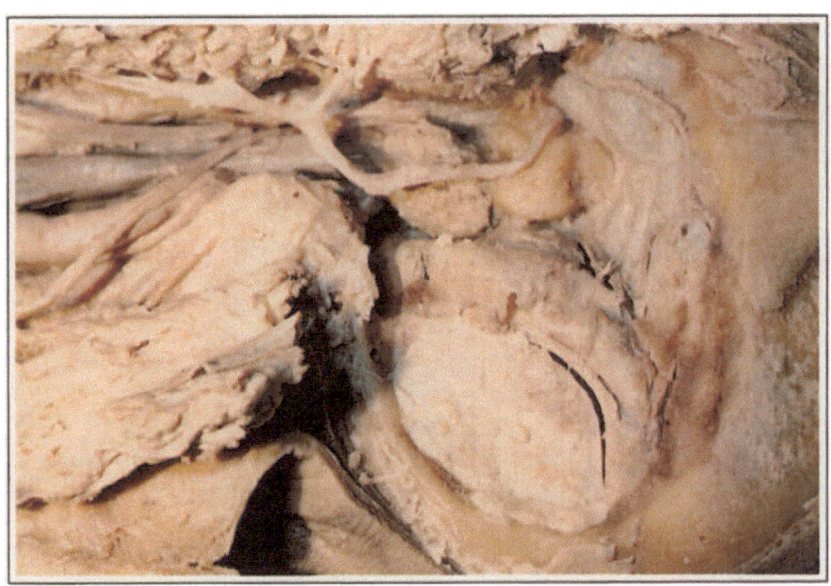

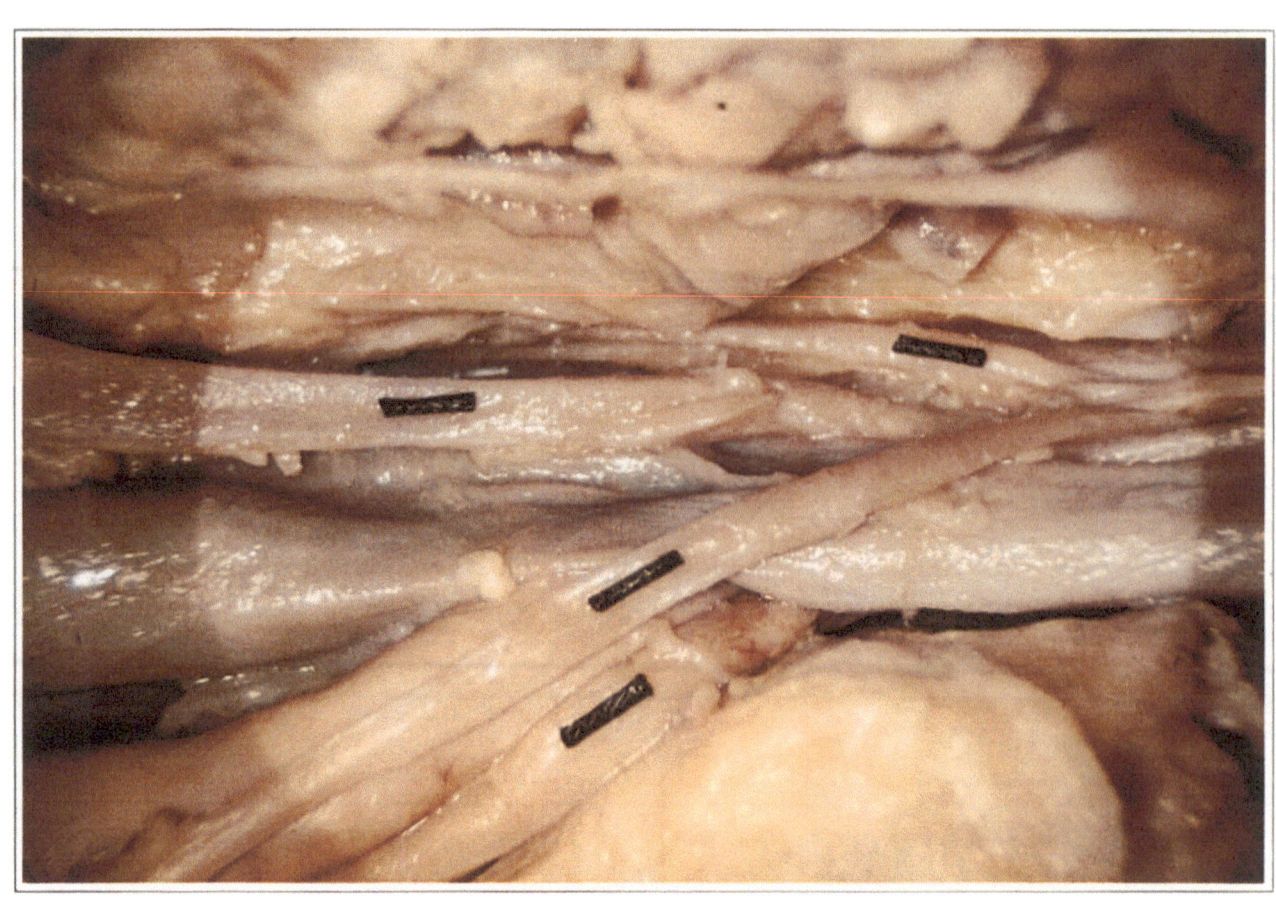

14. The carotid artery and cranial nerves IX, X, and XI are marked.

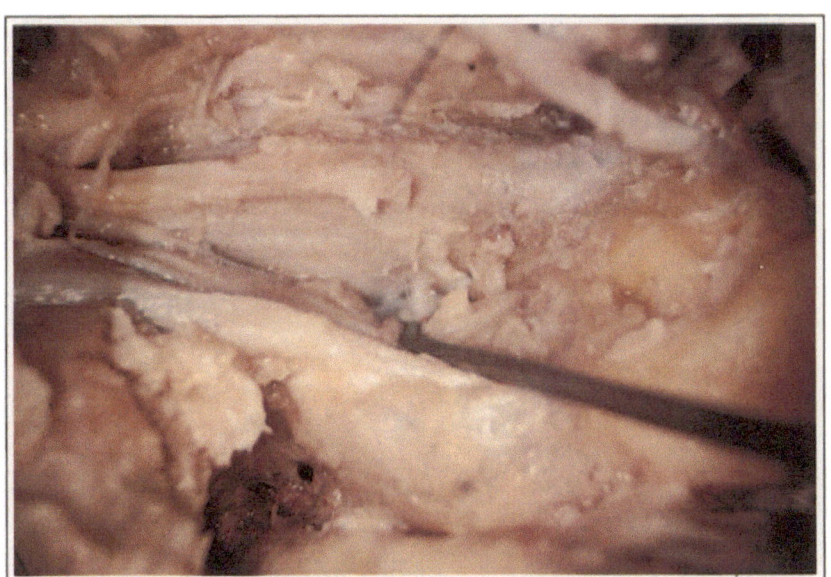

15. *The jugular bulb area.*

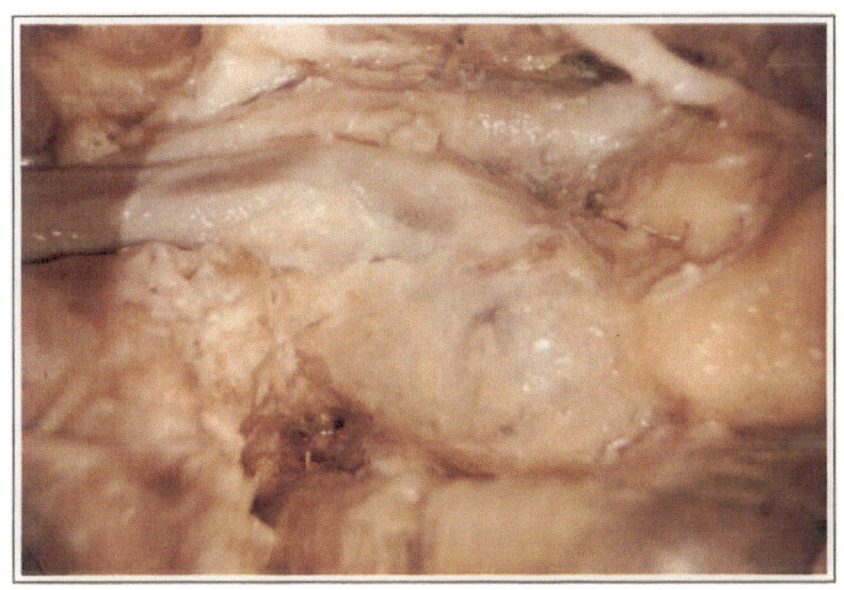

16. *The facial nerve (in the upper right), the carotid artery and jugular bulb are seen.*

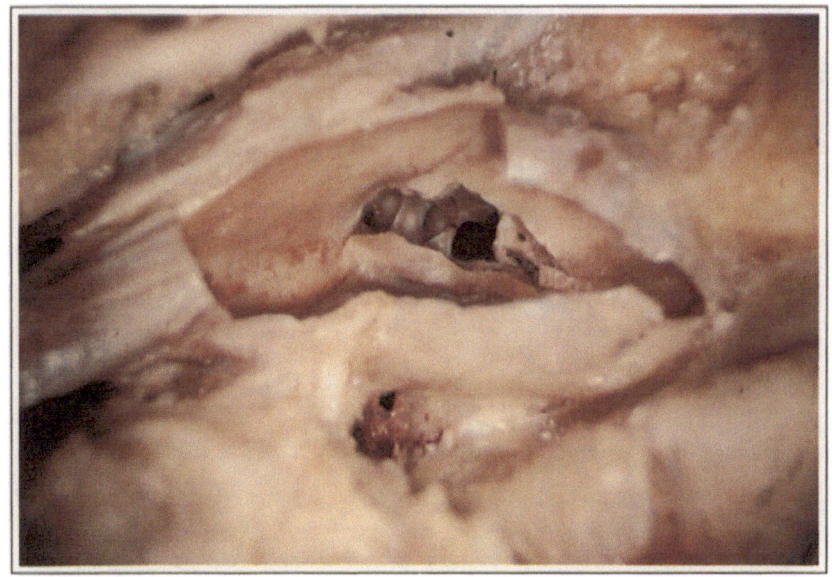

17. *The jugular bulb is opened demonstrating the entry of the inferior petrosal sinus.*

XII. SINGULAR NEURECTOMY

Section of the singular (posterior ampullary) nerve can be accomplished through a transtympanic approach. There is considerable risk to hearing with this procedure. The authors encourage surgeons who might perform this operation to use a postauricular approach to provide better exposure.

A. With the patient under general anesthesia, or under local anesthesia with sedation, a postauricular incision is made and the external auditory canal is transected.

B. A tympanomeatal flap is elevated and the middle ear entered. The EAC is enlarged posteriorly and superiorly so that the facial nerve, oval window (OW), and round window (RW) can be well visualized.

C. The round window niche is enlarged by removing the overhanging lip with a microdrill. This should provide access to the entire RW membrane.

D. The posterior semicircular canal ampulla lies just posterior and inferior to the RW membrane. This is also the origin of the singular canal which is 2-3 mm deep to the plane of the RW membrane. The singular nerve is most superficial near the posterior edge of the RW membrane.

E. Careful drilling just posterior and inferior to the edge of the RW membrane will reveal the white appearance of the myelinated singular nerve. A sharp hook is used to transect the nerve.

F. After sectioning the nerve, the depression in the bone is packed with absorbable gelatine sponge. The tympanomeatal flap and canal skin are returned to their normal locations and the post-auricular (PA) incision closed with absorbable suture.

Summary: *Disabling postural vertigo requiring surgery is not a common entity. For properly selected candidates, singular neurectomy can provide relief of symptoms. The patient must be made aware of the potential risk to auditory function. If the procedure is carried out under local anesthesia, the surgeon may monitor the success of the surgery by observing downbeating nystagmus with section of the nerve.*

11. ENDAURAL APPROACH (ONE)

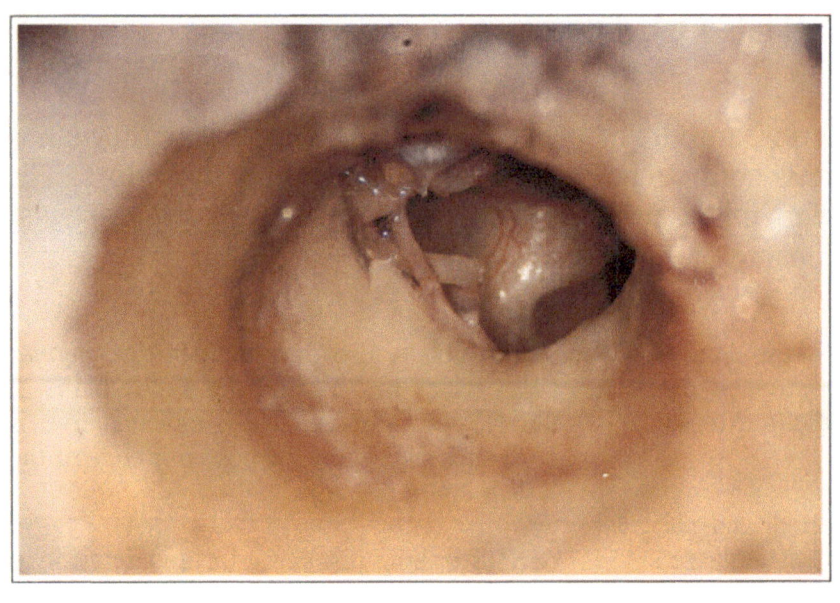

1. Through a postauricular (PA) approach, a tympano-meatal flap is elevated exposing the middle ear (ME).

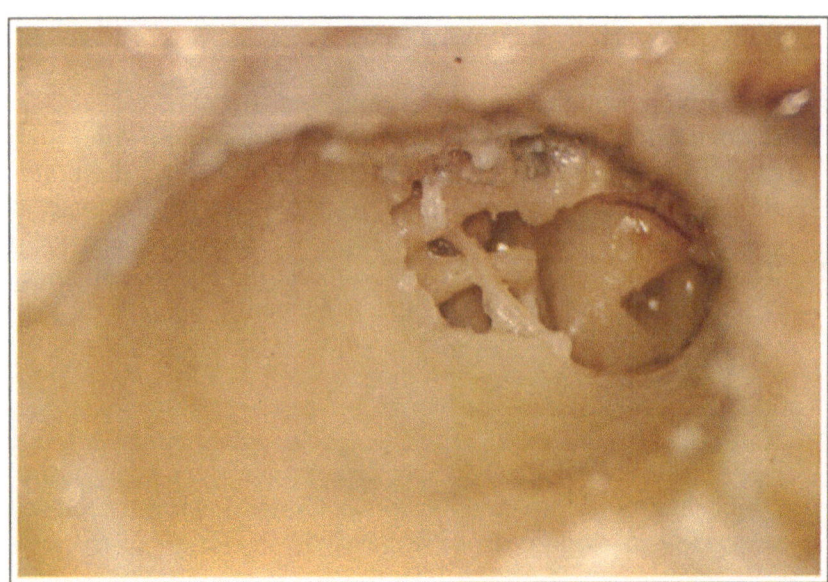

2. Exposure is facilitated by removing the posterior-superior canal wall.

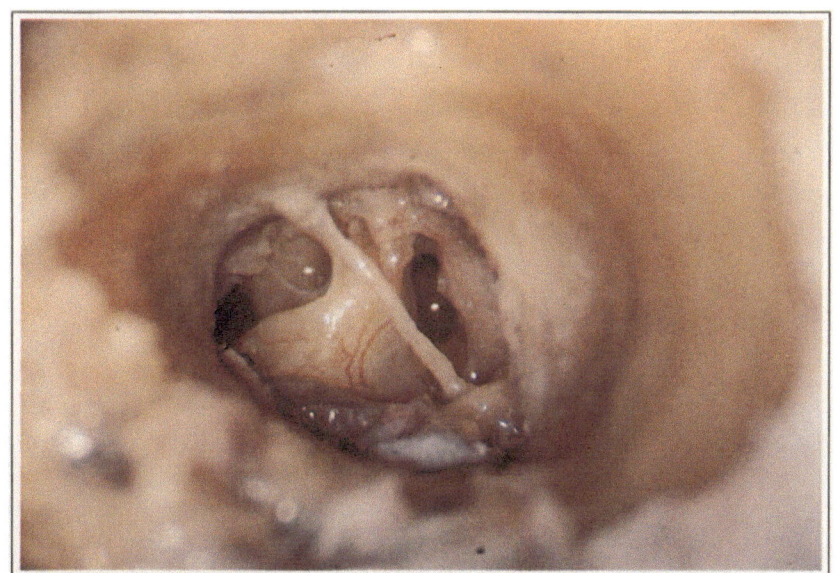

3. The incus and stapes are removed. This would not be done if hearing preservation were to be attempted.

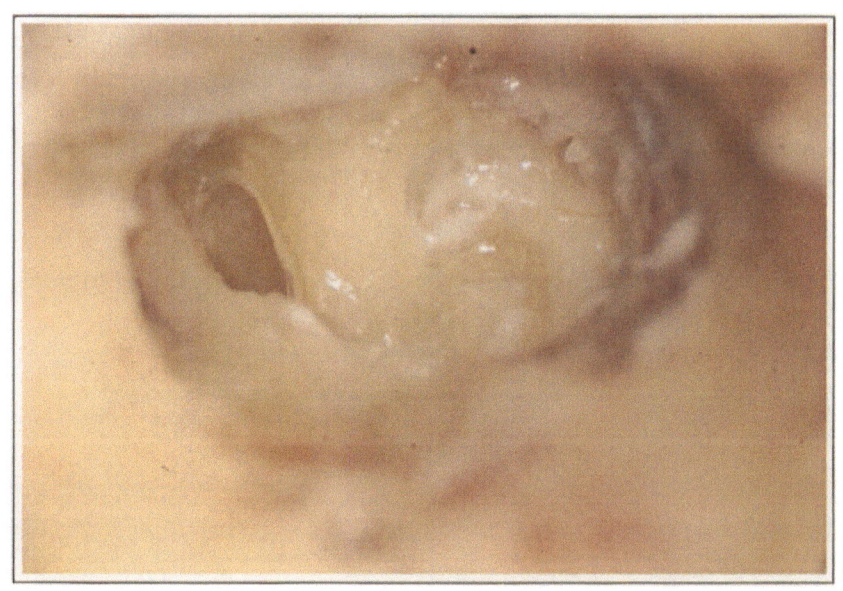

4. The lip of bone over the round window (RW) niche is drilled away, revealing the RW membrane.

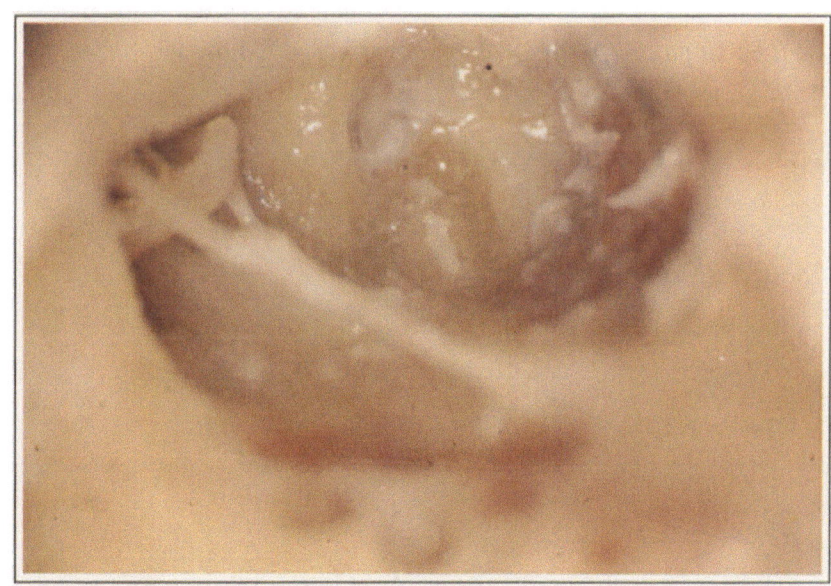

5. Posterior and inferior to the RW membrane, bone is drilled away to demonstrate the foramen singulare.

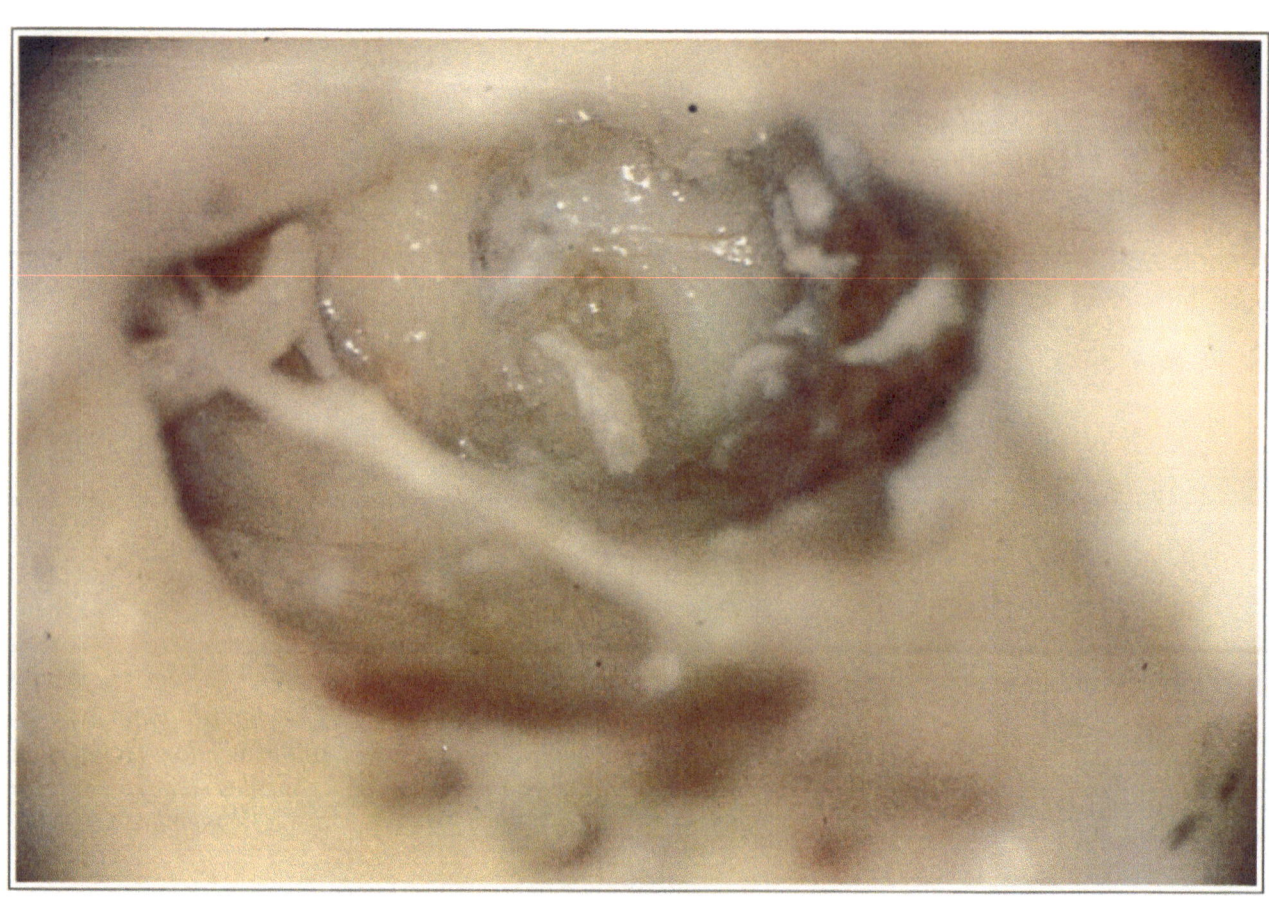

6. *The singular (posterior ampullary) nerve is now visualized.*

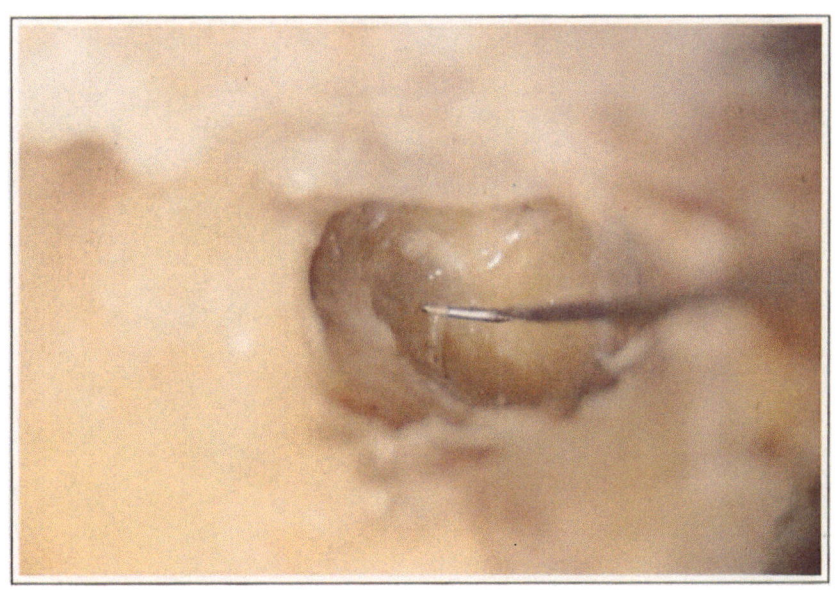

7. A sharp right angle hook transects the singular nerve.

8. Drilling too deep exposes the ampullated end of the posterior semicircular canal.

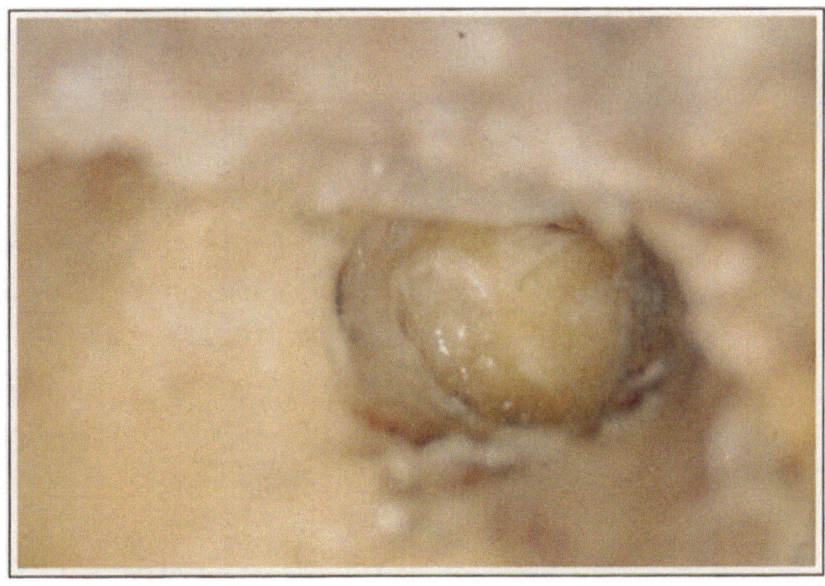

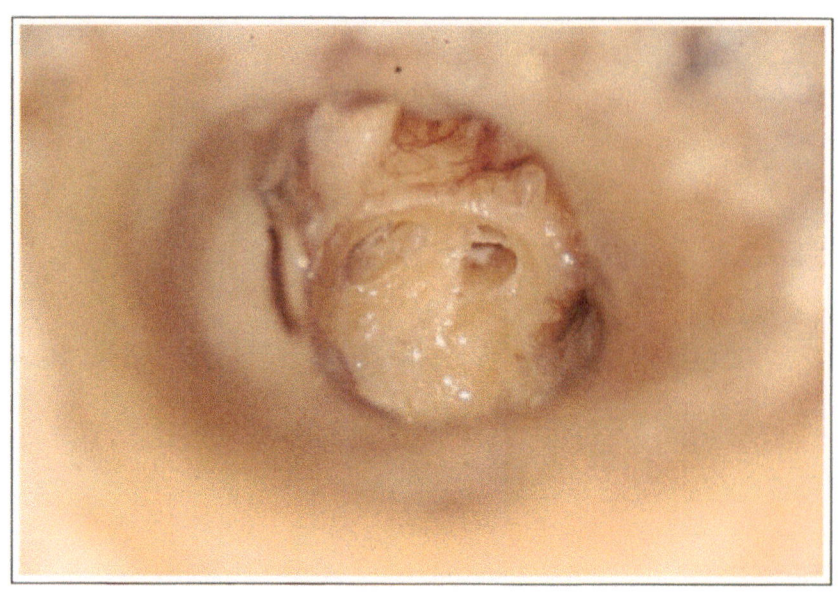

9. *Drilling forward and deep to the RW membrane exposes the cochlear turns.*

10. *Deeper dissection reveals the cochlear nerve.*

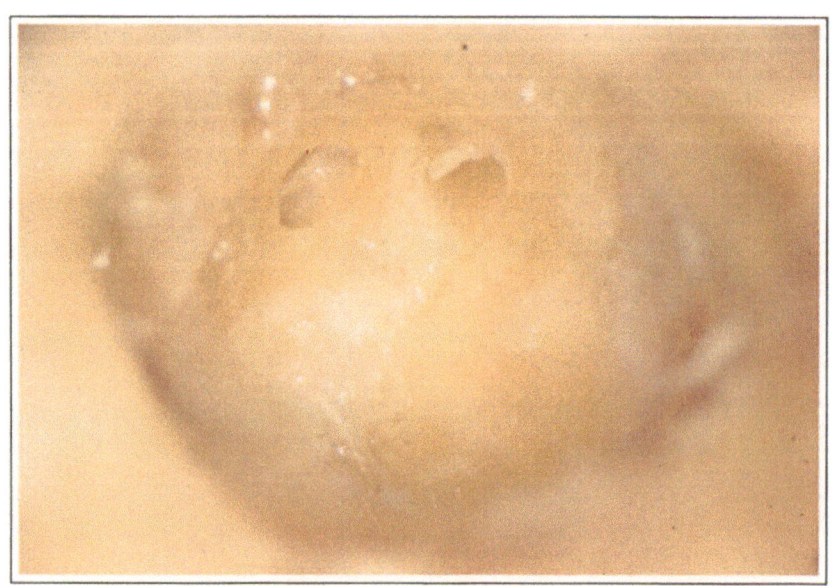

XIII. TRANSMEATAL OVAL WINDOW LABYRINTHECTOMY

Summary: *Transmeatal labyrinthectomy can be a highly effective means of ablating vestibular function. One must be diligent in one's search for neuroepithelium. If vestibular neuroepithelium is left behind, there is a high probability of failure. One must also take care not to injure the facial nerve during blind probing of the vestibule.*

A. A standard tympanomeatal flap is elevated, the middle ear space entered, and the posterior-superior canal wall removed to provide adequate exposure of the facial nerve and pyramidal eminence.

B. The incus and stapes are removed.

C. With a microdrill, the oval window (OW) and round window (RW) are connected. The basal turn of the cochlea is also widely opened.

D. Aspirate the saccule from the spherical recess and the utricle from the elliptical recess.

E. A 3 mm right angle hook is passed posteriorly and inferiorly to disengage the ampulla of the posterior semicircular canal. Pass the same hook posteriorly and superiorly to remove the ampullae of the superior and horizontal semicircular canals, taking care not to injure the facial nerve which may be dehiscent into the vestibule.

F. After thorough probing of the vestibule, pack the remaining recess with absorbable gelatine sponge that has been saturated with an ototoxic agent such as streptomycin or gentamycin.

G. The tympanomeatal flap is returned to its normal location and packed in place.

Summary: *Transmeatal labyrinthectomy can be a highly effective means of ablating vestibular function. One must be diligent in one's search for neuroepithelium. If vestibular neuroepithelium is left behind, there is a high probability of failure. One must also take care not to injure the facial nerve during blind probing of the vestibule.*

XIV. TRANSMEATAL COCHLEOVESTIBULAR NEURECTOMY

The transmeatal labyrinthectomy can be carried one step further to insure total vestibular ablation by opening the lateral end of the internal auditory canal (IAC) and sectioning the vestibular and cochlear nerves. This approach has disadvantages over the translabyrinthine approach in that the working space is quite limited and there is less anatomic definition of the neural contents of the IAC.

A. As with singular neurectomy, a postauricular incision is preferred for improved exposure. A tympanomeatal flap is elevated, the middle ear space entered, and the canal enlarged posteriorly for exposure of the facial nerve, RW, and OW.

B. The stapes and incus are removed. A microdrill connects the OW and RW and exposes the basal coil of the cochlea.

C. Identify the singular nerve and follow it toward the IAC. The posterior-inferior aspect of the IAC should be skeletonized without removing the transverse crest. The thin dura over the lateral end of the IAC should now be in view.

D. With a 1mm right angle hook open the dura. This maneuver transects the inferior vestibular nerve. The cochlear nerve can now be seen as a distinct nerve bundle entering the modiolus, and inferior to the facial nerve.

E. The superior vestibular nerve can usually be easily separated from the deeper lying facial nerve. The plane between these two nerves is developed with a sharp hook and the superior vestibular nerve sectioned.

F. A plug of adipose or temporalis muscle can be used to seal the end of the IAC. The middle ear should be filled with soft tissue also. The drum is replaced, the PA incision closed and a dressing applied.

Summary: *This approach to the contents of the IAC is quite restricted in its exposure. It places the facial nerve at greater risk as one has fewer familiar landmarks. The transmastoid, translabyrinthine approach to the IAC is the preferred surgical technique.*

12. ENDAURAL APPROACH (TWO)

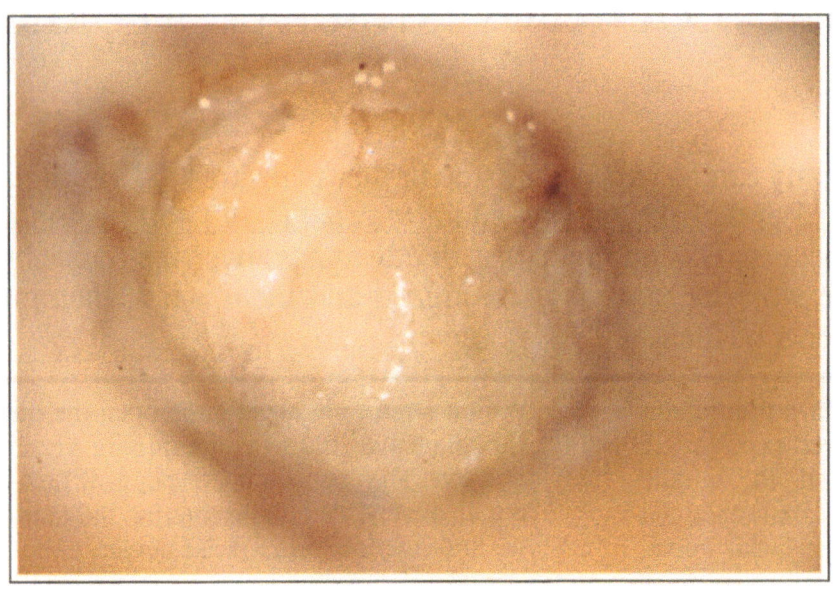

1. The OW and RW have been united by drilling between these two areas.

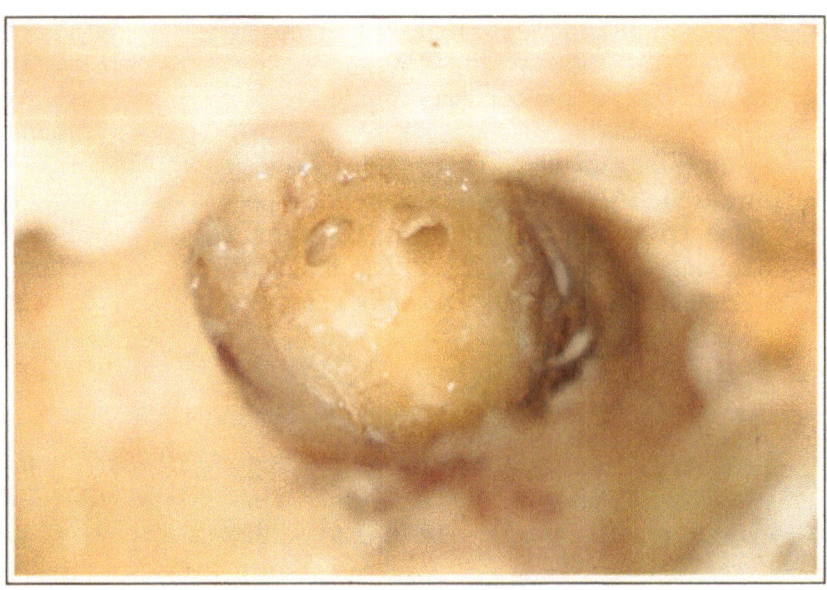

2. The cochlear turns and cochlear nerve are exposed by dissecting deeper.

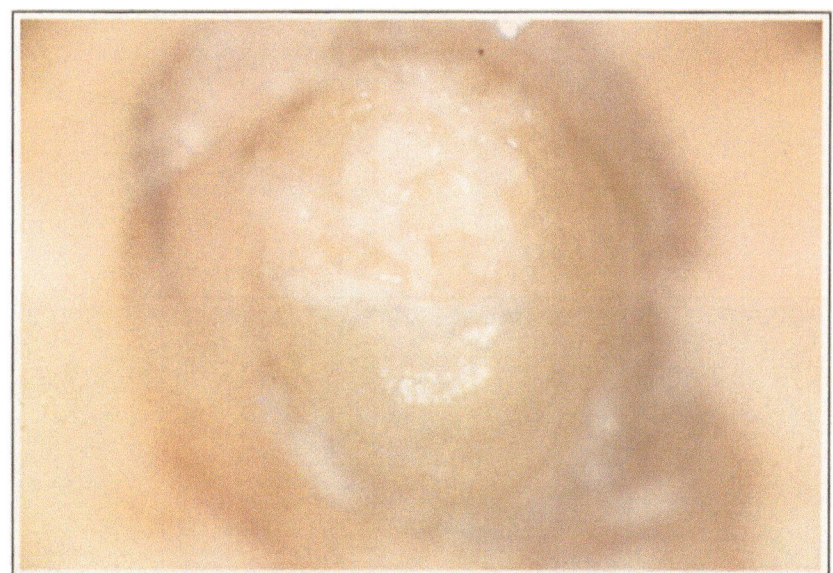

3. *By carefully thinning the bone superior and inferior to the cochlear nerve one exposes the dura of the internal auditory canal (IAC).*

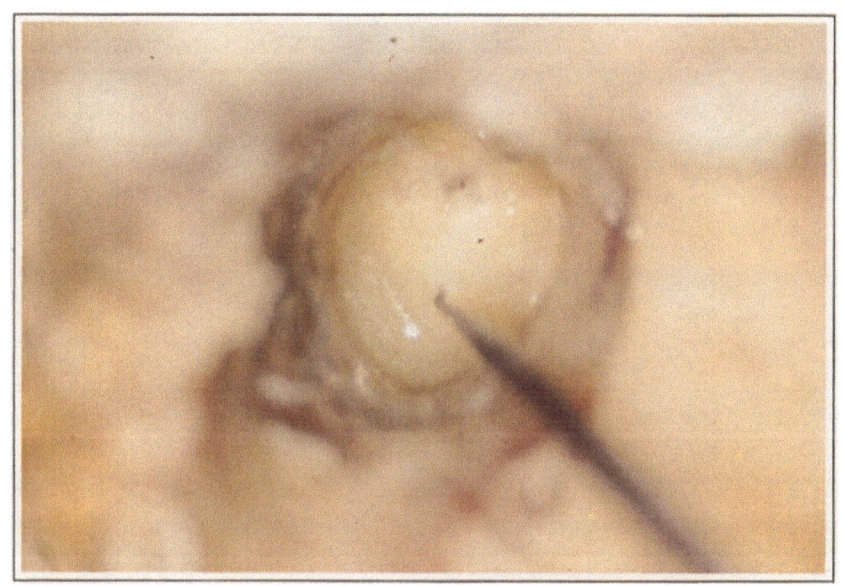

4. *The dura over the IAC is opened with a sharp hook.*

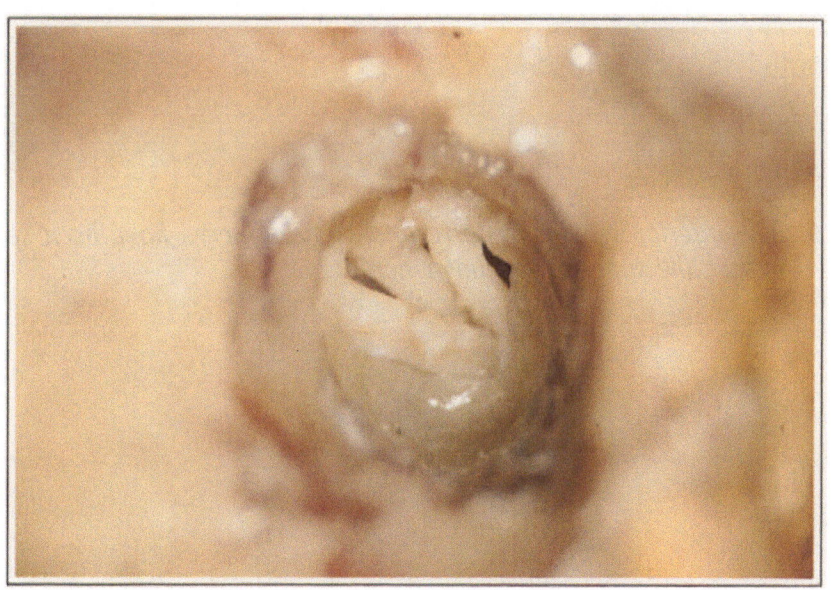

5. *The contents of the IAC are now well visualized.*

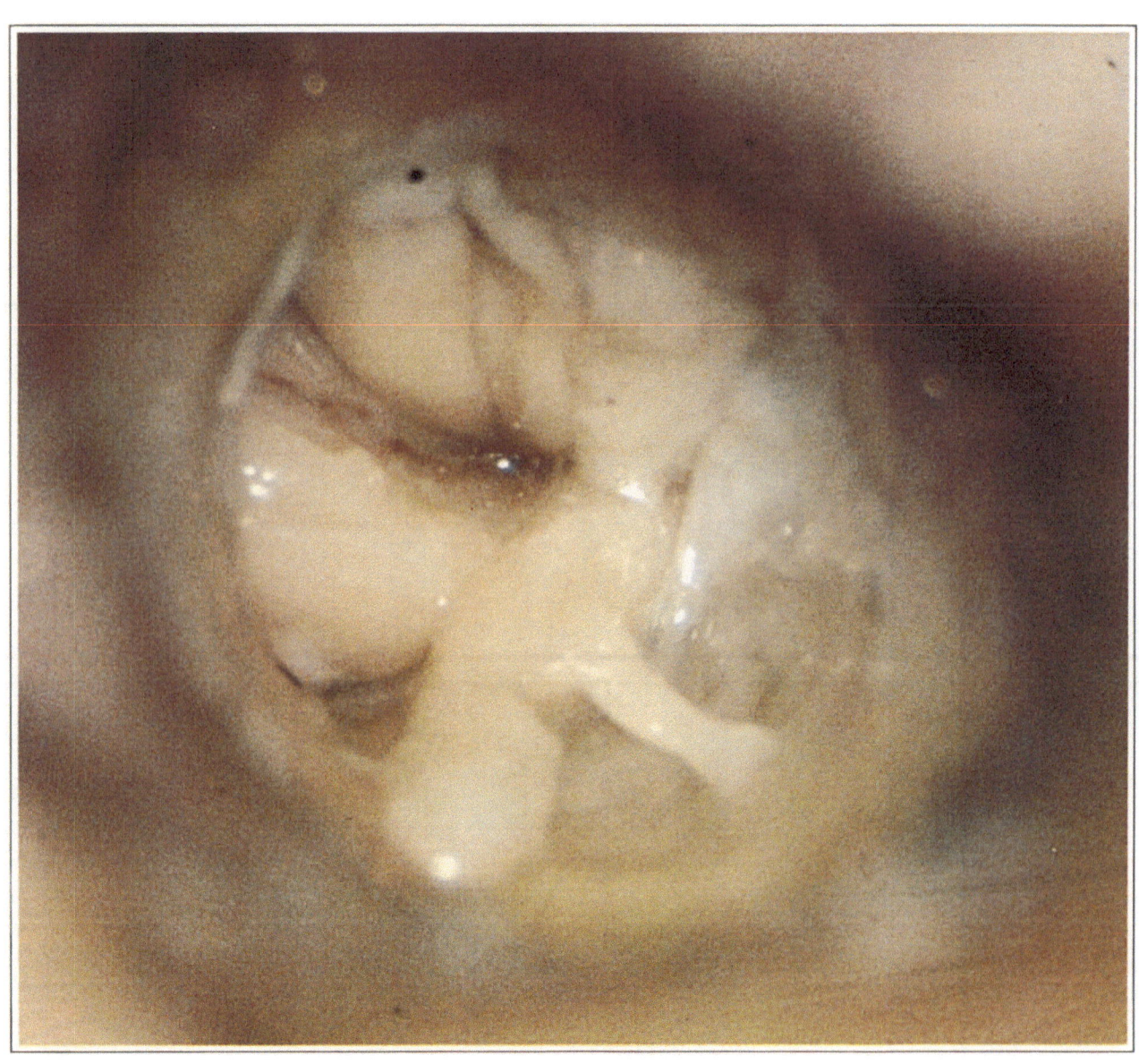

6. The inferior vestibular nerve and singular nerve have been sectioned and reflected posteriorly to expose the superior vestibular nerve.

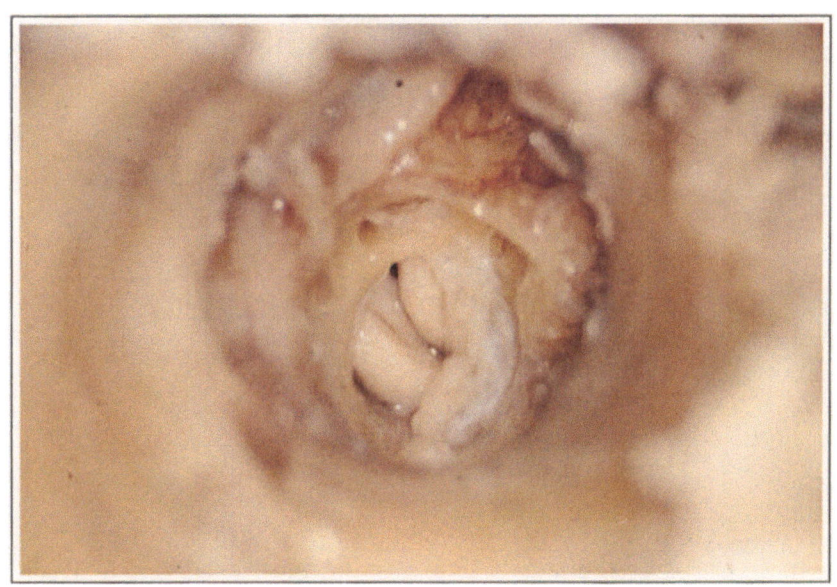

7. *Upward traction on the superior vestibular nerve demonstrates the plane between the facial and cochlear nerves.*

8. *The instrument points out the location of the facial nerve.*

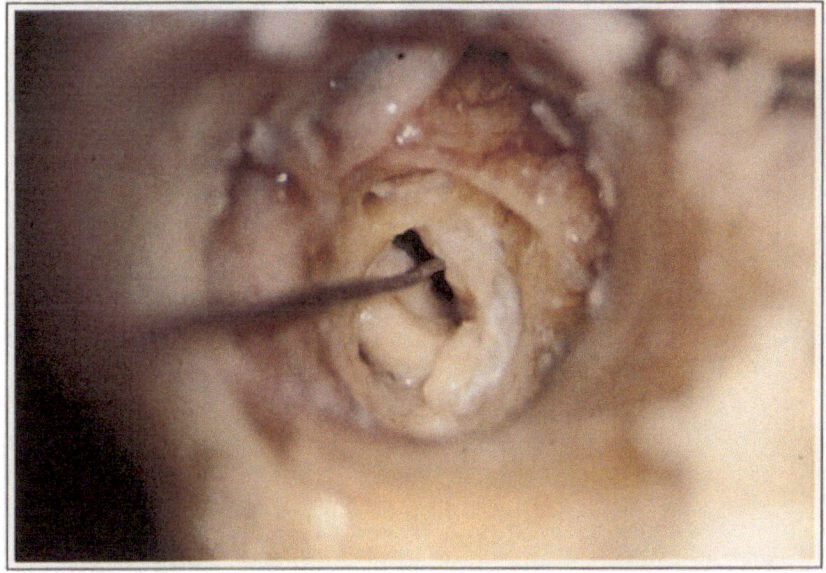

XV. FACIAL NERVE SURGERY

Proper identification and management of the facial nerve has been throughly discussed in the sections on translabyrinthine, transcochlear, infratemporal fossa, and middle fossa surgery. A brief review of the basic anatomy of the facial nerve and philosophical considerations will follow.

A. The otologic surgeon who endeavors to operate on the facial nerve must have the ability to perform both transmastoid and middle fossa surgery. The surgeon must also have familiarity with the extratemporal course of the facial nerve and be prepared to follow the nerve through the parotid compartment.

B. Following the mastoid course of the facial nerve first requires an adequate postauricular complete mastoidectomy. It is important to widely open the sinodural angle for increased access to the facial recess. In contracted mastoids, decompression of the sigmoid and posterior fossa dura may be necessary.

C. The retrofacial air tract should be widely opened. This is a very good place to positively identify the vertical portion of the facial nerve. It allows the surgeon to use the side of the burr and to take long strokes along the direction of the facial nerve, reducing the potential for injury.

D. The facial recess, or suprapyramidal recess, is next opened by saucerizing the posterior boney canal lateral to the course of the facial. Identify the course of the chorda tympani nerve and preserve this structure. Using progressively smaller burrs, the surgeon is able to open the air cells that are often found in the facial recess. These tracts can be followed into the middle ear. One should preserve the boney strut in the fossa incudis and take care not to touch the ossicular chain with the drill.

E. The facial recess is widened to expose the second genu of the facial nerve, the tympanic portion of the facial nerve, and the stapes and round window areas. One should also have good visualization of the cochleariform process.

F. As described earlier, decompression of the nerve is performed by leaving a thin shell of bone over the nerve while creating troughs on either side of the nerve. One should attempt to obtain at least 180 degrees of bone removal around the facial nerve. The remaining thin shell of bone over the nerve is removed with a dental excavator. The tympanic portion of the nerve is usually covered by a very thin layer of bone which is easily removed. Bone removal can be accomplished to the level of the geniculate ganglion.

G. If there is need to access the labyrinthine segment of the facial nerve, the approach that is selected depends upon the patient's auditory function. For patients that have total sensorineural loss in the affected ear, a translabyrinthine approach can be used. This is described in another section. Basically, this approach involves removing the labyrinth and skeletonizing the IAC. Bill's bar provides the key landmark identifying the entry of the facial nerve into the IAC. The entire facial nerve may be mobilized for resecting and grafting purposes by cutting the greater superficial petrosal nerve and rerouting the nerve posteriorly as described in transcochlear surgery.

H. For grafting the facial nerve, the greater auricular nerve is preferred. The graft is affixed with two or three sutures of 9.0 monofilament nylon sutures.

I. If access to the labyrinthine segment of the facial nerve is required and the patient has serviceable hearing, the surgeon must proceed with a middle fossa approach. The mastoid is left open for later reference and a standard middle fossa incision and dissection is begun. The greater superficial petrosal nerve is followed to the geniculate. The geniculate is uncovered with a diamond burr and the facial followed into the fundus of the IAC. Care is taken to avoid fenestrating the basal turn of the cochlea, the superior semicircular canal, and the vestibule. The IAC should be skeletonized as described earlier. The dura is opened to allow the surgeon to follow the facial nerve into the IAC. The epitympanum is carefully opened avoiding the head of the malleus. This will allow the surgeon to unite the transmastoid dissection with the middle fossa dissection. This will accomplish a total decompression/exposure of the intratemporal course of the facial nerve.

Summary: *In the case of trauma to the facial nerve, one may not know the extent of the injury preoperatively. In the event of a facial nerve neuroma, the margins of the lesion may not be delineated before surgery. Hence, the surgeon (and the patient) must be prepared to explore the entire course of the facial nerve by transmastoid, translabyrinthine, or middle fossa approaches.*

13. POSTAURICULAR TRANSMATOID APPROACH TO THE FACIAL NERVE

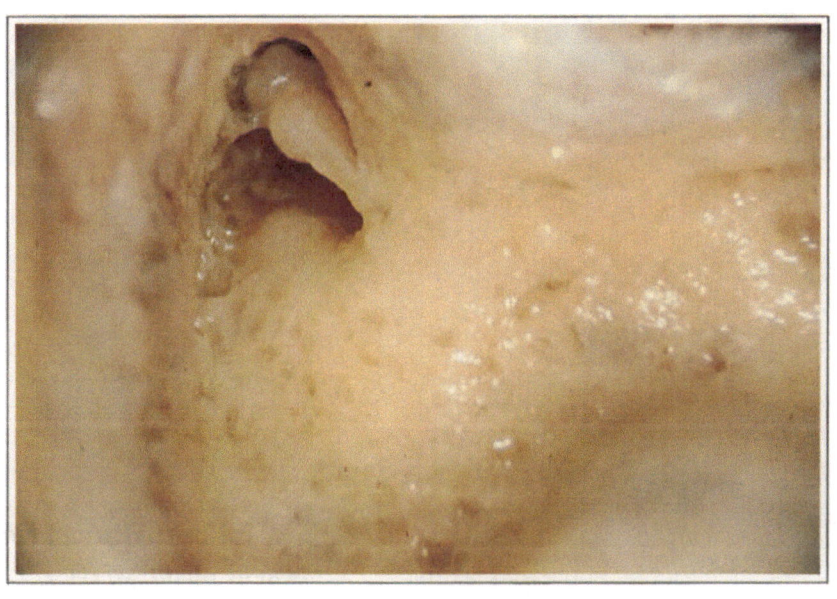

1. A complete mastoidectomy is performed, widely opening the epitympanum.

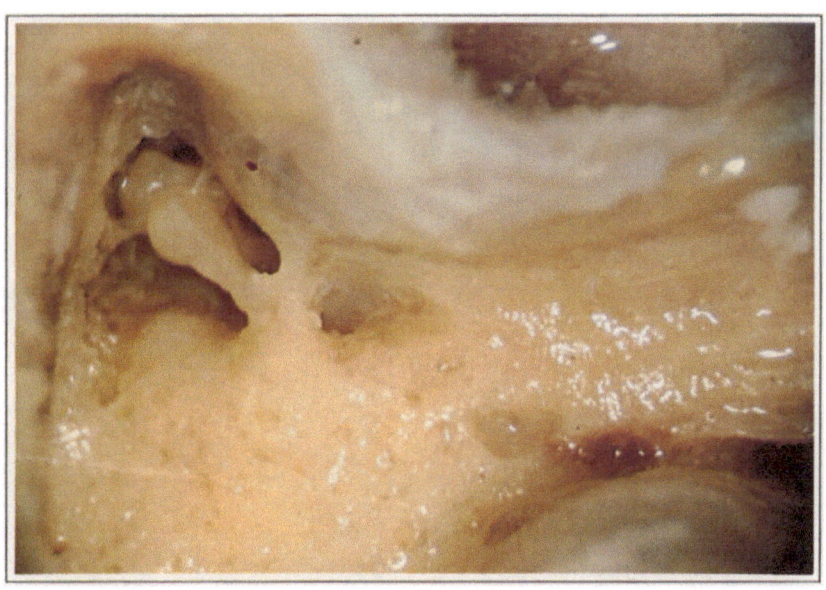

2. The facial recess is identified.

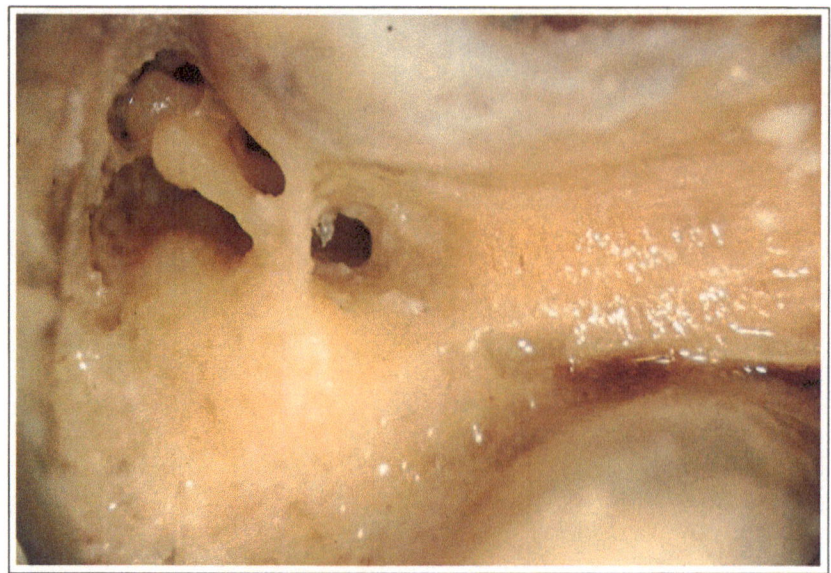

3. *Opening the facial recess.*

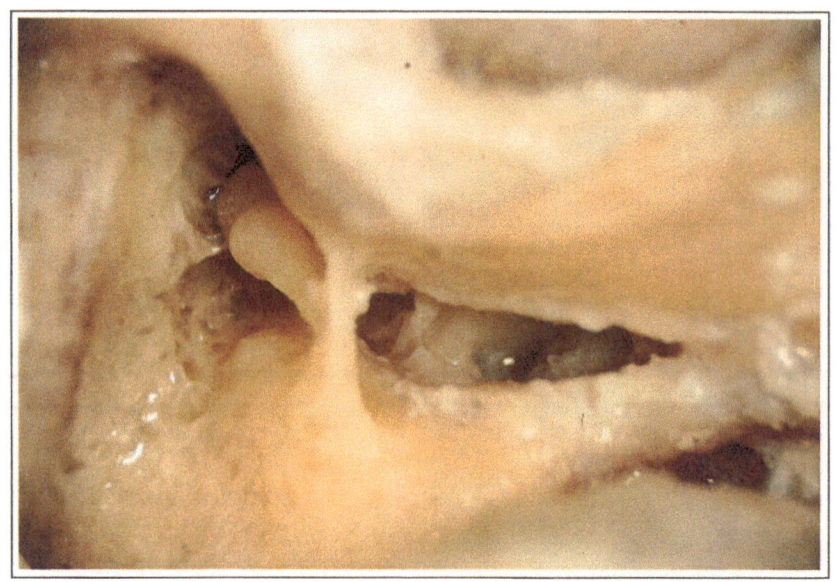

4. *Bone is removed around the mastoid facial nerve.*

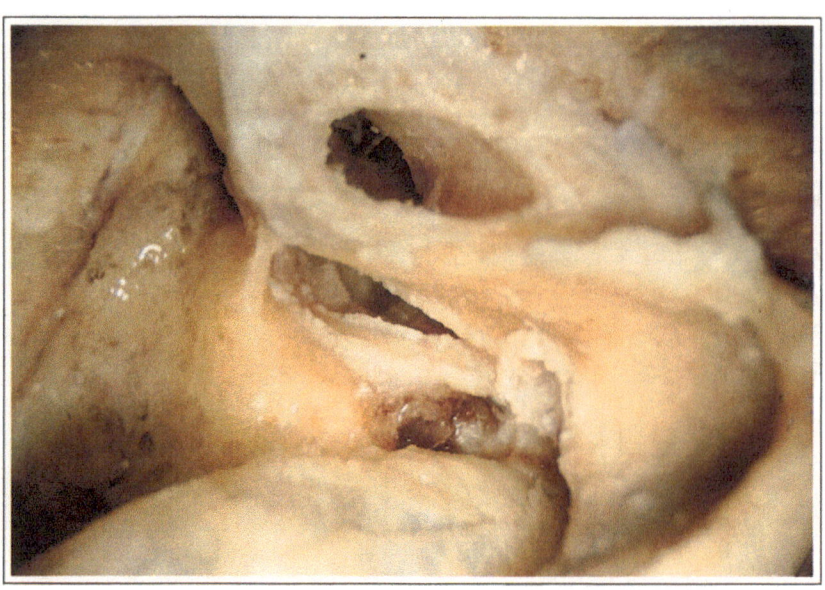

5. *The sheath is opened over the mastoid facial.*

100

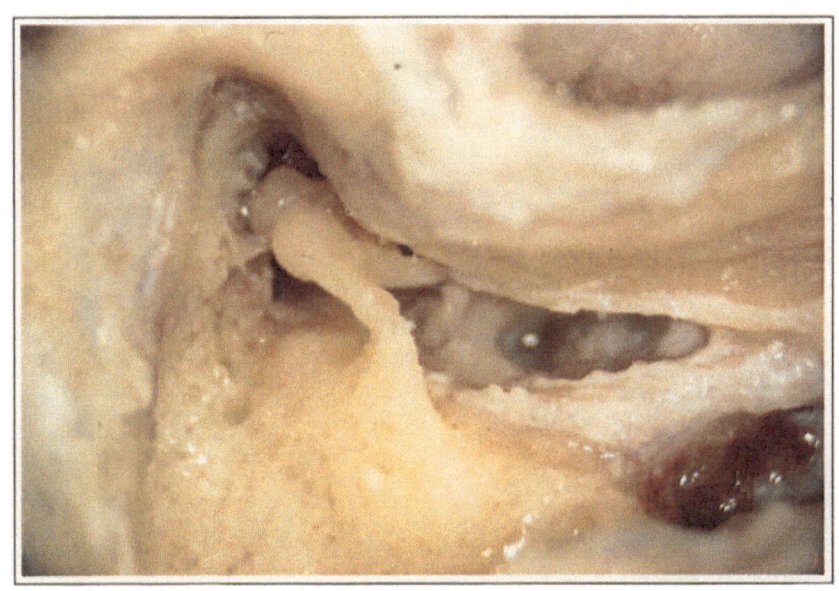

6. The bridge is removed. The tympanic facial is exposed.

7. The cochleariform process and COG are well visualized.

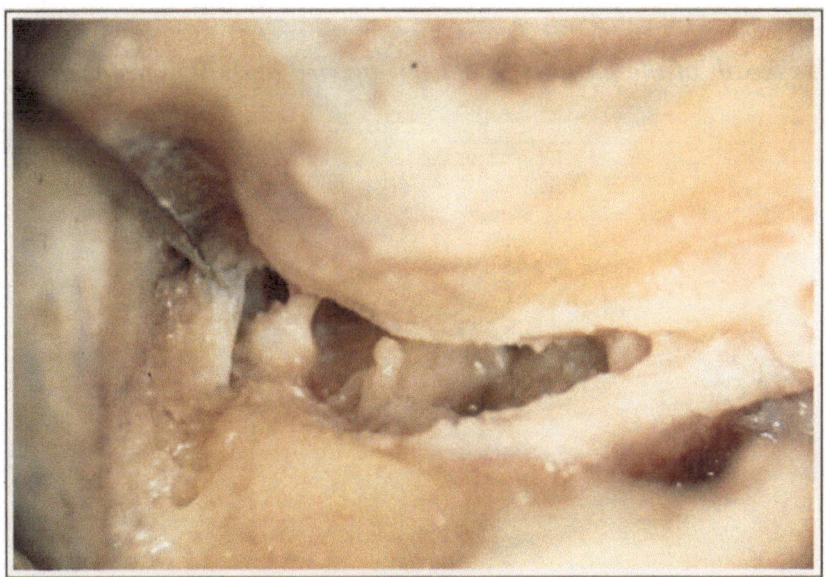

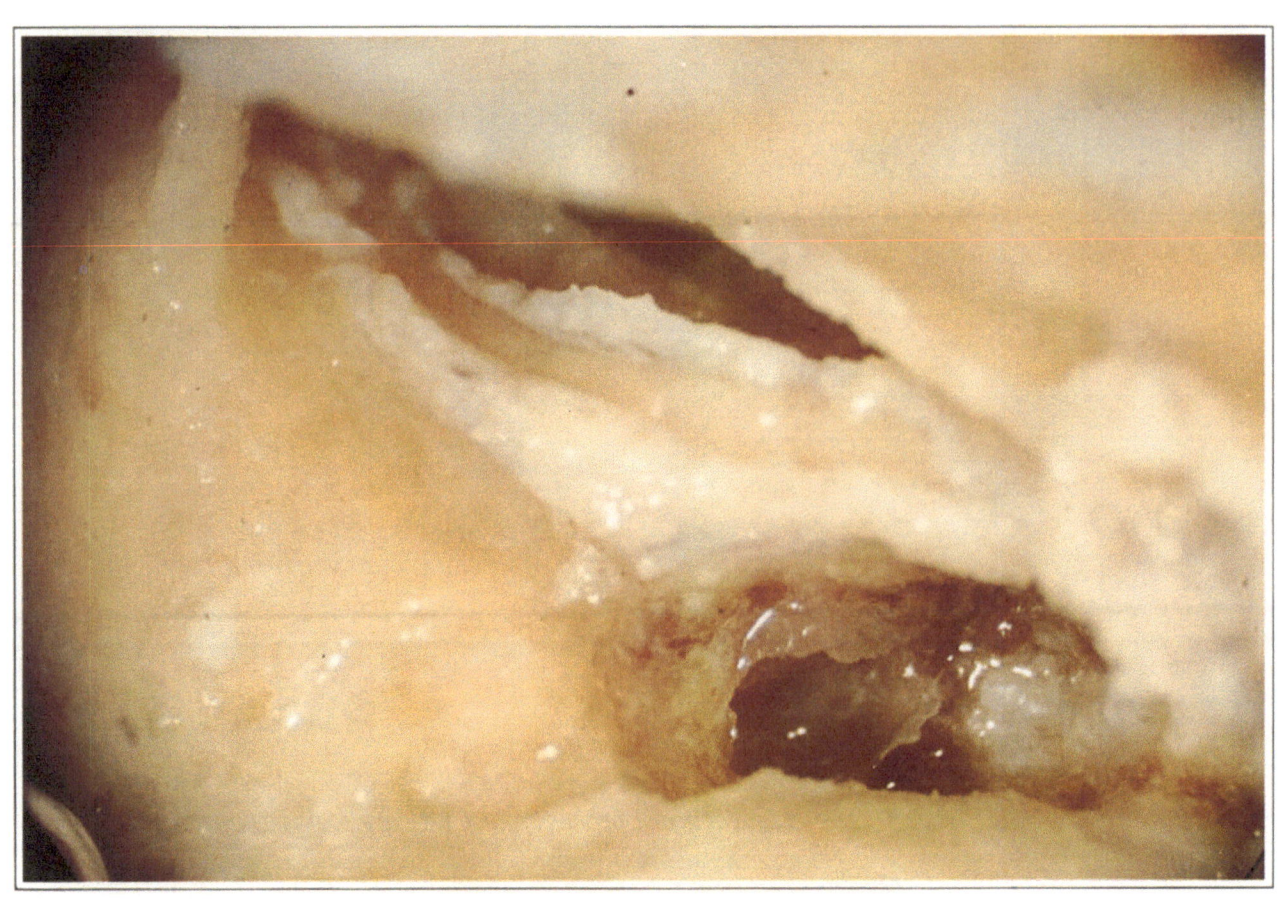

8. *The sheath of the facial is completely opened and the retrofacial air tract drilled.*

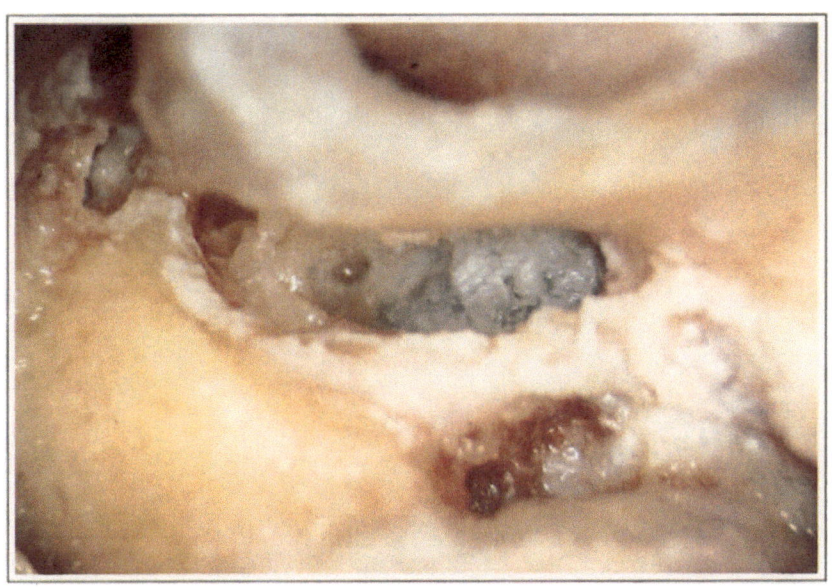

9. *The chorda tympani is sacrificed and the facial recess extended inferiorly.*

10. *The completed extended facial recess approach demonstrating the facial nerve at the stylomastoid foramen, hypotympanum, retrofacial area, and sac.*

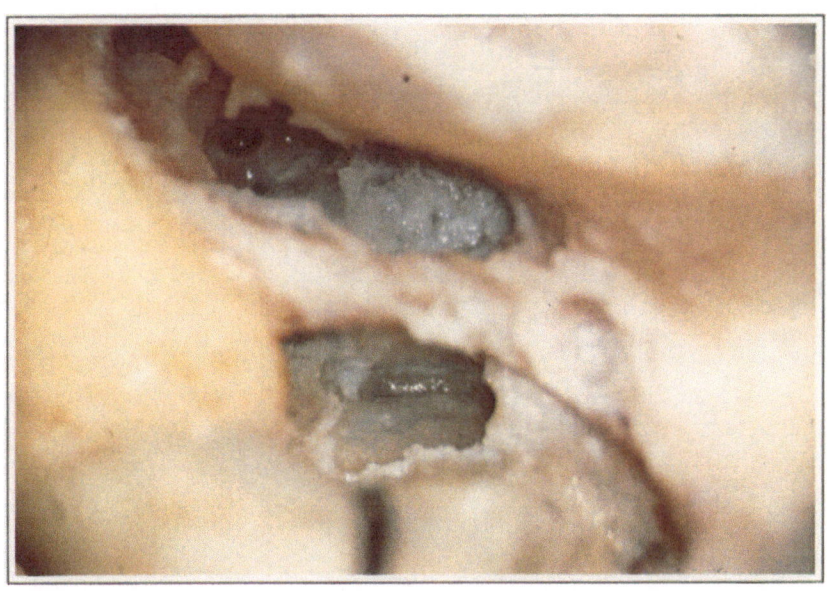

XVI. COMPLICATIONS OF OTO-NEUROSURGICAL PROCEDURES

A discussion of oto-neurosurgical procedures would be incomplete without a brief discussion of potential complications. It is not the authors' intent to describe in lengthy detail all aspects of oto-neurosurgical complications.

The complicated anatomy and difficult lesions involving the skull base and posterior fossa mandate precise pre-operative planning. Part of this planning involves adequately informing the patient and his family what is entailed in the particular surgery. Obviously, there is a fine line between informed consent and terrifying the patient. It is necessary that the patient be aware of the potential risks and hazards of the surgery about to be undertaken.

Anesthesia risks are often taken for granted. The risks and complications of general anesthetic should be outlined to the patient, especially in the case of unusual lesions such as catecholamine secreting paragangliomas where anesthetic management is particularly demanding.

Risk to the facial nerve varies with the type of surgery being performed. In the case where the facial nerve is to be rerouted, the patient must be prepared for the likely weakness that follows. The patient must be made aware of the possibility that the tumor invades or originates from the facial nerve, a situation that might require resection and grafting.

Cerebrospinal fluid leaks can occur following any oto-neurosurgical procedure. The patient must be aware, that if such a complication occurs, a secondary surgical procedure might be required. Of course, that chance of meningitis increases with the appearance of a CSF leak.

Postoperative infection may occur following oto-neurosurgical procedures and can take the form of a wound infection or intracranial infection such as meningitis. Such infections prolong hospitalization and introduce the possibility of antibiotic toxicity and allergic reactions. Any suspicion of a meningitis requires prompt investigation with a lumbar puncture.

Resection of large skull base tumors introduces the possibility of injury to cranial nerves IX, X, and XI with attendant problems of deglutition, phonation, and shoulder dysfunction. The possibility of tracheotomy needs to be discussed preoperatively.

The possibility of carotid artery compromise with resultant major neurologic deficits such as hemiparesis and aphasia needs attention preoperatively.

Eighth nerve consequences such as hearing loss, vertigo, and ataxia must be discussed with the patient.

Of course, each surgeon will have his or her manner of managing the possible consequences of surgery. In any event, today one can ill-afford to neglect a careful discussion of the risks, complications, expectations, and alternative forms of treatment with every patient.

Bibliography

1. Alvarez de Cozar F., Antoli Candela F.: Chirurgie trans vestibulaire. Rev. Laryng. Otol. Rhin. 1970; 91: 927-935

2. Arenberg I.K.: Results of endolymphatic sac to mastoid shunt surgery for Menière's disease refractory to medical therapy. Am. J. Otol. 1987; 8: 335-344

3. Arenberg I.K., Rask Andersen H., Wilbrand H., Stahle H.: The surgical anatomy of the endolymphatic sac. Arch. Otolaryng. 1977; 103: 1-11

4. Atkinson W.J.: Anterior inferior cerebellar artery: its variation, pontine distribution, and significance in surgery of the cerebellopontine angle tumors. J. Neurol. Neurosurg. Psychiatry. 1949; 12: 137-151

5. Belal A. Ylikoski J.: Pathology as it relates to ear surgery II. Labyrinthectomy. J. Laryng. Otol. 1983; 97: 1-10

6. Benecke J.E.Jr., House H.P.: Glomus tumor: forty-year follow-up on a patient treated with surgery and radiation.Otolaryngol. Head Neck Surg. 1988; 98: 92-94

7. Brackman D.E., Hitselberger W.E.,: Retrolabyrinthine approach technique and newer indications. Laryngoscope. 1987; 88: 286-297

8. Brackman D.E., Hitselberger W.E., Robinson J.V.: Facial nerve repair in cerebellopontine angle surgery.Ann. Otol. Rhinol. Laryngol.1978; 87: 772-777

9. Bretlau P., Thomsen J., Tos M.. Jonsen N.J.: Placebo effect in surgery for Menière's disease: a three-year follow-up study of patients in a double blind placebo controlled study on endolymphatic sac shunt surgery. Am. J. Otol.1984; 5: 558-561

10. Calbucci F. Tognetti F. Bollini C. Cuscini A. Michelucci R. Tassinari C. A.: Intracranial microvascular decompression for "cryptogenic" hemifacial spasm, trigeminal and glossopharyngeal neuralgia, paroxismal vertigo and tinnitus: I. Surgical tecnique and results. Ital. J. Neurol. Sci. 1986; 7: 359-366

11. Cawthorne T.: Membranous labyrinthectomy via the oval window for Menière's disease. J. Laryngol. Otol. 1957; 71: 524-527

12. Colletti V., Fiorino F.G., Sittoni V., Carlisle L.: Chemical labyrinthectomy with NaCl: Menière's disease treatment with apposition of NaCl in the vestibule. Acta Otolaryngol. (Stock) 1987; 104: 7-12

13. Cushing H.: Tumors of the nervus acusticus and the syndrome of the cerebellopontine angle. Philadelphia, W.B. Saunders Co., 1977

14. Dandy W.E.: An operation for the total removal of cerebellopontine (acoustic) tumors. Surg. Gynecol. Obstet. 1925; 41: 129-148

15. Dandy W.E.: Treatment of Menière's disease by section of only the vestibular portion of the acoustic nerve. Bull. Johns Hopkins Hosp. 1933; 53: 52-55

16. Desgeorges M., Sterkers J.M.: Surgery of large neurinomas of the acoustic nerve performed only by the translabyrinthine approach. Apropos of 50 cases. Neurochirurgie 1984; 30: 355-364

17. Eckermeier L., Pirsig W., Mueller D.: Histopathology of 30 non-operated acoustic schwannomas. Arch. Otorhinolaryngol. 1979; 222: 1-9

18. Eiras J., Gomez J., Carcavilla L.: Suboccipito-transmeatal microsurgical approach in giant acoustic neuromas. Results in 12 consecutive cases. Neurochirurgie 1984; 30: 17-24

19. Fisch U.: Carotid lesions at the skull base. In: Brackmann D.E. (Ed.) *Neurological surgery of the ear and skull base*. New York, Raven Press, 1982

20. Fisch U.: Infratemporal fossa approach for extensive tumors of the temporal bone and base of skull. In: Silverstein H. (Ed.) *Neurological Surgery of the Ear*. Birmingham, Aesculapius Publishing Co., 1977

21. Fisch U.: Infratemporal fossa approach for glomus tumors of the temporal bone. Ann. Otol. Rhinol. Laryngol. 1982; 91: 474-479

22. Fisch U.: Infratemporal fossa approach to tumors of the temporal bone and base of the skull. J.Laryngol. Otolaryngol. 1978; 92: 949-967

23. Fisch U.: The infratemporal fossa approach for nasopharyngeal tumors. Laryngoscope 1983; 93: 36-44

24. Fischer G., Morgon A., Fischer C., Bret P., Massini B., Kzaiz M., Charlot M.: Complete excision of acoustic neurinoma. Preservation of the facial nerve and hearing. Neurochirurgie 1987; 33: 169-183

25. Frerebeau P., Benezech J., Uziel A., Coubes P., Segnarbieux F., Malonga M.: Hearing preservation after acoustic neurinoma operation. Neurosurgery 1987; 21: 197-200

26. Friberg U., Jansson B., Rask-Andersen H., Bagger-Sjoback D.: Variations in surgical anatomy of the endolymphatic sac. Arch. Otolaryngol. Head Neck Surg. 1988; 114: 389-394

27. Gacek R.R.: Singular neurectomy update. Ann. Otol. Rhinol. Laryngol. 1982; 91: 469-473

28. Gacek R.R.: Transection of the posterior ampullary nerve for the relief of benign paroxysmal positional vertigo. Ann. Otol. Rhinol. Laryngol.1974; 83: 596-605

29. Gantz B., Fisch U.: Modified transotic approach to the cerebellopontine angle. Arch. Otolaryngol. 1983; 109: 252-256

30. Garcia-Ibanez E., Garcia-Ibanez J.I.: *Chirurgia del conducto auditivo interno.* Madrid, F.Garcia Sicilia, 1973

31. Gardner G., Robertson J.H., Clark W.C., Bellott A.L.Jr., Hamm C.W.: Acoustic tumor management-combined approach surgery with CO2 laser. Am. J. Otol. 1983; 5: 87-108

32. Gibson W.P.: A study of endolymphatic sac surgery. The results after reconstructing the sac versus those in operations that failed to open the lumen and satisfactorily insert a silastic implant. Otolaryngol. Clin. North Am. 1983; 16: 181-188

33. Glasscock M.E., Dickins J.R.E.: Complications of acoustic tumor surgery. Otolaryngol. Clin. North Am. 1982; 15: 883-896

34. Glasscock M.E., Harris P.F., Newsome G.: Glomus tumors: diagnosis and treatment. Laryngoscope 1974; 84: 2006-2032

35. Glasscock M.E., Hay J.W., Jackson C.G., Steenerson R.L.: A one-stage combined approach for the management of large cerebellopontine angle tumors. Laryngoscope 1978; 88: 1563-1576

36. Glasscock M.E., Kveton J.F., Jackson C.G., Levine S.C., McKennan K.X.: A systematic approach to the surgical management of acoustic neuroma. Laryngoscope 1986; 96: 1088-1094

37. Glasscock M.E., Miller G.W., Drake F.D., Kanok M.M.: Surgery of the skull base. Laryngoscope 1978; 8: 905-923

38. Glasscock M.E.III, Dickens J.R.E., Wiet R.J.: Preservation of hearing in acoustic tumor surgery middle fossa technique. In: *Neurological Surgery of the Ear*, vol.2, New York, Aesculapius Publishers Inc., 1979

39. Glasscock M.E.III, Jackson C.G., Withaker S.R.: The argon laser in acoustic tumor surgery. Laryngoscope 1981; 91: 1405-1416

40. Goin D.W., Rasband R.W., Mischke R.E., Weaver M.: Endolymphatic sac surgery in Mondini's dysplasia: a report of 16 cases. Laryngoscope 1984; 94: 343-347

41. Graham M.D., Kemink J.L.: Surgical management of Menière's disease with endolymphatic sac decompression by wide bony decompression of the posterior fossa dura: technique and results. Laryngoscope 1984; 94: 680-683

42. Graham M.D., Kemink J.L.: Transmastoid labyrinthectomy: surgical management of vertigo in the nonserviceable hearing ear. A five-year experience. Am. J. Otol. 1984; 5: 295-299

43. Gvelesiani A.O., Makhmudov U.B., Blagoveshchenskaia N.S., Dobrovolskii G.F.: Topographo-anatomic basis of the translabyrinthine approach to the internal auditory canal and the cerebellopontine angle. Zh. Vopr. Neirokhir. 1986; 2: 20-26

44. Hitselberger W.E., House W.F.: A combined approach to the cerebellopontine angle: a suboccipital-petrosal approach. Arch. Otolaryngol. 1966; 84: 267-285

45. Hitselberger W.E., Pulec J.L.: Trigeminal nerve (posterior root) retrolabyrinthine selective section: operative procedure for intractable pain. Arch. Otolaryngol. 1972; 96: 412-415

46. Hou J.H.: Suboccipital transmeatal approach for microsurgical removal of acoustic neuroma. Chung Hua I Hsueh Tsa Chih. 1983; 63: 670-672

47. House W.F.: Long-term results of endolymphatic subarachnoid shunt surgery in Menière's disease. In: Shambaugh G.E., Shea J.J. (Eds.) *Shambaugh International Workshop on Middle Ear Microsurgery and Fluctuant Hearing Loss, 5th*, Northwestern University Medical School, Alabama, 1976: Proceedings; Huntsville, Strode Publishers, 1977; 441-444

48. House W.F.: Subarachnoid shunt for drainage of endolymphatic hydrops: a preliminary report. Laryngoscope 1962; 72: 713-729

49. House W.F.: Surgical exposure of the internal auditory canal and its contents through the middle cranial fossa. Laryngoscope 1961; 71: 1363-1365

50. House W.F., De La Cruz A.: Transcochlar approach to the petrus apex and clivus. Trans. Am. Acad. Ophtalmol. Otolaryngol. 1977; 74: 927-931

51. House W.F., De La Cruz A., Hitselberger W.E.: Surgery of the skull base: Transcochlear approach to the petrous apex and clivus. Otolaryngology 1978; 86: 770-779

52. House W.F., Gardner G., Hughes R.L. et al.: Middle cranial fossa approach. Arch. Otolaryngol. 1968; 88: 631-641

53. House W.F., Hitselberger W.E.: The transcochlear approach to the skull base. Arch. Otolaryngol. 1976; 102: 334-342

54. House W.F., Luetje C.M. (Eds.): Acoustic Tumors, Vol.1, Baltimore, University Park Press, 1979

55. House W.F., Luetje C.M. (Eds.): Acoustic Tumors, Vol.2, Baltimore: University Park Press, 1979

56. Huang T.S., Lin C.C.: Endolymphatic sac surgery for Menière's disease: a composite study of 339 cases. Laryngoscope 1985; 95: 1082-1086

57. Jackler R.K., Luxford W.M., Brackmann D.E., Monsell E.M.: Endolymphatic sac surgery in congenital malformations of the inner ear. Laryngoscope 1988; 98: 698-704

58. Jackson C.G.: Skull base surgery. Am. J. Otol. 1981; 3: 161-171

59. Jannetta P.J., Møller M.B:, Møller A.R.: Disabling positional vertigo. N.Engl. J.Med. 1984; 310: 1700-1705

108

60. Jannetta P.J., Møller A.R., Møller M.B.: Technique of hearing preservation in small acoustic neuromas. Ann. Surg. 1984; 200: 513-523

61. Jannetta P.J., Møller M.B., Møller A.R., Sekhar L.N.: Neurosurgical treatment of vertigo by microvascular decompression of the eighth cranial nerve. Clin. Neurosurg. 1986; 33: 645-665

62. Jenkins H.A., Fisch U.: The transotic approach to resection of difficult acoustic tumors of the cerebellopontine angle. Am. J. Otol. 1980; 2: 70-76

63. Jiang D.J.: Surgical treatment of 224 cases of big acoustic neurinoma with special consideration on 76 cases treated microsurgically. No Shinkei Geka 1985; 13: 1175-1180

64. Kartush J.M., Telian S.A., Graham M.D., Kemink J.L.: Anatomic basis for labyrinthine preservation during posterior fossa acoustic tumor surgery. Laryngoscope 1986; 96: 1024-1028

65. Kasantikul V., Netsky M.G., Glasscock M.E.III, Hays J.W.: Acoustic neurilemmoma: Clinicoanatomical study of 103 patients. J.Neurosurg. 1980; 52: 28-35

66. Kitahara M., Kitajima K., Yazawa Y., Uchida K.: Endolymphatic sac surgery for Menière's disease: eighteen years experience with the Kitahara sac operation. Am. J. Otol. 1987; 8: 283-286

67. Kudo T., Ito K.: Microvascular decompression of the eighth cranial nerve for disabling tinnitus without vertigo: a case report. Neurosurgery 1984; 14: 338-340

68. Lehrer J.F., Quraishi A.U., Poole D.C.: The role of endolymphatic sac surgery in the management of secondary endolymphatic hydrops associated with perilymphatic fistulas: preliminary observations. Am. J.Otol. 1987; 8: 93-95

69. Mazzoni A. et al.: *La chirurgia del condotto uditivo interno.* Ferrara, SATE, 1977

70. Mejier E., Hoogland G.A.: Suboccipital (retrosigmoidal) approach for cerebellopontine angle tumours. Adv. Otorhinolaryngol. 1984; 34: 143-149

71. Meyerhoff W.L.: Surgical section of the posterior ampullary nerve. Laryngoscope 1985; 95: 933-935

72. Michelucci R., Tassinari C.A., Samoggia G., Tognetti F., Calbucci F.: Intracranial microvascular decompression for "cryptogenic" hemifacial spasm, trigeminal and glossopharyngeal neuralgia, paroxysmal vertigo and tinnitus: II. Clinical study and long-term follow up. Ital. J. Neurol. Sci. 1986; 7: 367-374

73. Millen S.J., Meyer G.: Retrosigmoid intracanalicular vestibular nerve section: an alternative surgical approach for Menière's disease. Am. J. Otol. 1986; 7: 330-332

74. Miyamoto R.T., Althaus S.R., Wilson D.F., Brookler K.H.: Middle fossa surgery. Report of 153 cases. Otolaryngol. Head Neck Surg. 1985; 93: 529-535

75. Morrison A.W.: Cochleostomy or endolymphatic sac surgery for advanced Menière's disease. Otolaryngol. Clin. North Am. 1983; 16: 135-142

76. Nely J.G.: Gross and microscopic anatomy of the eighth cranial nerve in relationship to the solitary schwannoma. Laryngoscope 1981; 91: 1412-1531

77. Olivecrona H.: The removal of acoustic neurinomas. J.Neurosurg. 1967; 26: 100-103

78. Paparella M.M., Hanson D.G.: Endolymphatic sac drainage for intractable vertigo (method and experiences). Laryngoscope 1976; 86: 697-703

79. Pillsbury H.C., Arenberg I.K., Ferraro J., Ackley R.S.: Endolymphatic sac surgery. The Danish sham surgery study: an alternative analysis. Otolaryngol. Clin. North Am. 1983; 16: 123- 127

80. Pluchino F., Fornari M., Luccarelli G.: Intracranial repair of interrupted facial nerve in course of operation for acoustic neurinoma by microsurgical technique. Acta Neurochir. (Wien) 1986; 79: 87-93

81. Portmann G.: Surgical treatment by opening the saccus endolymphaticus. Arch. Otolaryngol. 1927; 6: 309-319

82. Portmann M.: The Internal Auditory Meatus-Anatomy, Pathology and Surgery. Edinburgh, Churchill Livingstone, 1975

83. Portmann M., Sterkers J.M., Charchon R., Chouard C.H.: *Le conduit auditif interne (anatomie, pathologie, chirurgie).* Paris, Librairie Arnette, 1973

84. Pulec J.L.: Labyrinthectomy: Indications, technique, and results. Laryngoscope 84: 1552-1573

85. Rhoton A.L.Jr.: Microsurgical anatomy of acoustic neuromas. Neurol. Res. 1984; 6: 3-21

86. Rhoton A.L.Jr.: Microsurgical anatomy of the brainstem surface facing an acoustic neuroma. Surg. Neurol. 1986; 25: 326- 339

87. Romanenko D.A.: Anatomy of the facial nerve canal with regard to microsurgery of the ear. Vestn. Otorinolaringol. 1985; 2: 36- 40

88. Rutka J.A., Nedzelski J.M., Barber H.O.: Results of endolymphatic sac surgery for Menière's disease. J. Otolaryngol. 1984; 13: 70-72

89. Sakaki T., Morimoto T., Miyamoto S., Kyoi K., Utsumi S., Hyo Y.: Microsurgical treatment of patients with vestibular and cochlear symptoms. Surg. Neurol. 1987; 27: 141-146

90. Samii M.: Facial nerve grafting in acoustic neurinoma. Clin. Plast. Surg. 1984; 11: 221-225

91. Samii M., Penkert G.: Results of 110 microsurgical acoustic neuroma operations. Eur. Arch. Psychiatry Neurol. Sci. 1984; 234: 42-47

92. Samii M., Turel K.E., Penkert G.: Management of seventh and eighth nerve involvement by cerebellopontine angle tumors. Clin. Neurosurg. 1985; 32: 242-272

93. Sanna M., Zini C., Mazzoni A., Gandolfi A., Pareschi R., Pasanisi E., Gamoletti R.: Hearing preservation in acoustic neuroma surgery. Middle fossa versus suboccipital approach. Am. J. Otol. 1987; 8: 500-506

94. Sato K., Shimoji T., Yaguchi K., Sumie H., Kuru Y., Ishii S.: Middle fossa arachnoid cyst: clinical, neuroradiological and surgical features. Childs Brain 1983; 10: 301-316

95. Sato O., Tanabe S., Sohma T.: Microsurgical technique of posterior fossa trasmeatal approach for acoustic neurinoma- preservation of facial and cochlear nerves. No Shinkei Geka 1984; 12: 779-784

96. Savary P., Charissoux G.: Surgical opening of the endolymphatic sac in Menière's disease; our experience from 1962- 1980. J. Otolaryngol. 1984; 13: 73-75

97. Savic D., Djeric D.: Intratemporal operative paralysis of the facial nerve. Rev. Laryngol. Otol. Rhinol. (Bord) 1987; 108: 239- 244

98. Schuknecht H.F., Hammerschlag P.E.: Transcanal labyrinthectomy. In: Silverstein H., Norell H. (Eds.) *First Symposium on Neurological Surgery of the Ear*. Birmingham, Ala, Aesculapius Press 1977

99. Silverstein H.: Transmeatal labyrinthectomy with and without cochleovestibular neurectomy. Laryngoscope 1976; 86: 1777-1791

100. Silverstein H., Norrel H.: Neurological surgery of the ear. Birmingham, Alabama, Aesculapius Publishing Company, 1977

101. Silverstein H., Norrel H.: Retrolabyrinthine surgery: a direct approach to the cerebellopontine angle, Otolaryngol. Head Neck Surg. 1980; 88: 462-465

102. Silverstein H., Norrel H., Hyman S.M.: Simultaneous use of CO2 laser with continuous monitoring of eighth cranial nerve action potential during acoustic neuroma surgery. Otolaryngol. Head Neck Surg. 1984; 92: 80-84

103. Silverstein H., Smouha E., Jones R.: New microsurgical instruments for retrosigmoid posterior fossa internal auditory canal surgery. Otolaryngol. Head Neck Surg. 1988; 98: 262-265

104. Smith M.F., Lagger R.L.: Hearing conservation in acoustic neurilemmoma surgery via the retrosigmoid approach. Otolaryngol. Head Neck Surg. 1984; 92: 168-175

105. Spector G.J., Smith P.G.: Endolymphatic sac surgery for Menière's disease. Ann. Otol. Rhinol. Laryngol. 1983; 92: 113-118

106. Sterkers J.M., Sterkers O., Maudelonde C., Corlieu P.: Preservation of hearing by the retrosigmoid approach in acoustic neuroma surgery. Adv. Otorhinolaryngol. 1984; 34: 187-192

107. Szekely T.: Surgery of glomus tumors. HNO 1984; 32: 54-58

108. Tarlov E.C.: Microsurgical vestibular nerve section for intractable Menière's syndrome; technique and results. Clin. Neurosurg. 1986; 33: 667-684

109. Thomsen J., Bretlau P., Tos M., Johnsen N.J.: Endolymphatic sac-mastoid shunt surgery. A nonspecific treatment modality? Ann. Otol. Rhinol. Laryngol. 1986; 95: 32-35

110. Wade P.J., House W.: Acoustic neuromas: middle fossa approach-hearing preservation. Otolaryngol. Head Neck Surg. 1984; 92: 184-193

111. Wigand M.E., Haid T., Berg M., Rettinger G.: Microsurgical neurolysis of the 8th cranial nerve in cochleo-vestibular disorders using an extended transtemporal approach. HNO 1983; 31: 295-302

112. Winkler D., Nowak G., Freckmann N.: Convulsive tic in combination with vertigo attacks and their surgical treatment by microvascular decompression. Nervenarzt 1987; 58: 47-48

113. Wright J.W., Hicks G.W.: Valved implants in endolymphatic sac surgery. Am. J. Otol. 1987; 8: 307-312

114. Yamane H., Igarashi M.: Free-floating cells in the endolymphatic sac after surgical utricular nerve section. ORL J. Otorhinolaryngol. Relat. Spec. 1984; 46: 289-293

115. Zemskaia A.G., Bersnev V.P., Rogulov V.A.: Neurinomas of the acoustic nerve in childhood and adolescence. Zh.Vopr. Neirokhir 1984; 6: 7-12

116. Zini C., Sanna M.: La timpanotomia posteriore nel trattamento chirurgico delle otomastoiditi croniche. In: *Dissertationes de aurium partis mediae morbis*. XX Conventus Societas rhino-laringologica latina 1974

117. Zini C., Sanna M., Jemmi G., Gandolfi A.: Transmastoid extralabyrinthine approach in traumatic facial palsy. Am. J. Otol. 1985; 6: 216-221

Subject Index